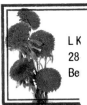

MW01122667

Suck It Up Sunshine

sands press

Brockville, Ontario

Suck It Up Sunshine

by Megan McIntyre

sands press

sands press

A division of 3244601 Canada Inc.
300 Central Avenue West Brockville, Ontario
K6V 5V2

Toll Free 1-800-563-0911 or 613-345-2687
http://www.sandspress.com
ISBN 978-1-988281-22-3

Copyright © Megan McIntyre 2016
Cover Concept by Kristine Barker
Formatting by Renee Hare
Publisher Kristine Barker, Sands Press

This book is a memoir. It reflects the author's present recollections of experiences over time. Some names and characteristics have been changed, some events have been compressed, and some dialogue has been recreated.

1st Printing Spring 2017
To book an author for your live event, please call: 1.800.563.0911

Submissions

Sands Press is a literary publisher interested in new and established authors wishing to develop and market their product. For more information please visit our website at www.sandspress.com.

Dedications & Thanks

To Karen Wright for showing me girls can do anything they put their minds to!

To Anita Minov for helping navigate the writing process.

To Ben Guyatt for leading the way to becoming an author.

To Perry, Kristine and the Sands Press team for believing that my story was worth telling.

To my family for being by my side throughout the writing process.

Author's Note

This book is written in the style of a memoir. I bared my soul on each and every page.

The characters are based on real people in my life. The names have been changed for legal reasons.

To allow for better flow, the timelines have been squished together and in some cases rearranged to suit the narrative.

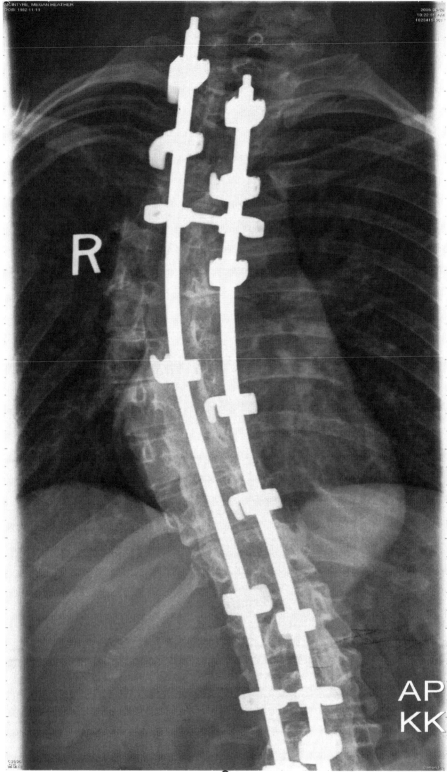

Preface

I've always liked writing whether in the form of a journal or free verse poetry. Open-ended topics are my favorite kind of writing because I prefer not to count syllables. Once I finished formal education, I picked any topic that I wished to write about.

One could say I broke the mold when I came out of the womb. I'm not one to colour inside the lines so to speak. Medically speaking, I'm what doctors refer to as abnormal. I have Friedreich's Ataxia (F. A.), a nerve disorder affecting my balance, among other things. I don't like the title. I don't fancy being anyone, but myself. I'll go into more detail later on. I'm not going to live under a label. So I'm disabled; I'm a human being first and foremost. My name is Megan.

My older brothers, Will and Chad, were raised in the same household, yet we are all unique. My Dad talked about how before having kids he had three theories about raising children. After raising three kids, his theories went out the window. At the end of the day, we are all bonded together as a family.

Although handicap parking and accessible washrooms are requirements, I can't dwell on them. Life should be lived to your fullest potential. I try to be a positive person and not let the things I can't do takeover my conscious mind. I'll be the one in the parking spot by the door.

Writing is therapeutic for me. A good friend told me to write what I know. Since my life is somewhat unusual, my story makes for an interesting plot line. Frankly, I'm just being me.

From a young age, I liked to make lists and plan for my future. At age fourteen, I was diagnosed with Friedreich's Ataxia and my whole life flashed before me. It shattered, like a broken mirror. Unfortunately, I can't choose not to be disabled. I can, however, decide how I will react when I hit a speed bump in the road of life.

I'm not going to lie. Some days do suck. Future events become

1

foggy and fate plucks your life plan from your hands. Our existence is a lot like a 'Choose Your Own Adventure' book. I'm dating myself. If you don't recall this type of novel, look up the book series next time you're at the library. Depending on the path you choose, the story changes.

I think of myself as flexible and to a certain degree that's true. The rest of the time I'm more of a type A person. I'd rather be in control of the situations around me. I suppose that isn't too surprising because my mother was a primary teacher and my Dad was an elementary school principal. Both jobs required management. I'm fond of the term leadership, as opposed to a control freak.

My Mom is ever the teacher. As a small child, she'd point a building out because there is never a bad time for a learning experience. Even as an adult, she'll state the significance of a statue. I used to get irritated when she expanded my knowledge. I realize my Mom couldn't shut off the teacher inside of herself. Secretly, I've grown to look forward to her educational moments.

Whether you're disabled or not life is a game of choices. Some people will peak in high school, while other friends will run a relatively smooth course. Some people are quietly fighting an invisible illness, while outwardly their life appears to be close to perfection.

We should all be nicer to the mathletes and nerdy types, because you never know with whom you'll spend your life. In high school, the oddest student I could think of was Christian Ruthers. I didn't have to worry about potentially marrying him because he later came out as gay. My gaydar was seriously off-kilter.

Every day I woke up and chose to be happy. Some days I found being upbeat difficult and I ended up having a down day. Other days I would be in high spirits from start to finish.

When I began writing, I established a routine of a specific time and place where I would let myself dream. I didn't know if my writing was good, bad, or indifferent. My mentor paved the way for me to be able to produce the best work I possibly could.

My story became a diary for me. I've never kept a daily journal on the computer, but I'm good at recalling dates and events from the past. I remember stuff that isn't remarkable like when I last wore my navy top. Working on the computer means that I can go back and edit until the writing is just the way I'd like it to be.

When I write, being a perfectionist works in my favour. If I completed a piece of work that didn't meet my personal standards, I wouldn't be happy with the finished product. A rewrite of a chapter or editing a book seems like a massive undertaking. When my work is completed, I'm satisfied my writing is the best I could create.

My zodiac sign is 'Scorpio', which means I don't do anything without passion being behind me. I utilize the creativity in my mind to my benefit.

I'm Megan McIntyre and this is my story. Laugh, cry and smile. Sit back and buckle up and prepare for a ride on the roller coaster that is my life.

Firsts

Did my doctor just tell me to "Suck it up Sunshine."? I can't believe his words. Judging by the faces of the medical students behind him, I didn't misunderstand him. Dr. Sutton is my neuromuscular doctor. He's probably the only person who could tell me to suck it up and get away with it. My parents were expecting me to react negatively to his statement instead I didn't say a peep.

At one of my semi-annual appointments, I had asked him if he could surgically alter my winged shoulder that resulted from my curved spine. Dr. Sutton's remarks made me pause and reflect. I took a deep breath and sucked up my emotions prior to moving forward. There'll be more on him later.

I was dealt a shitty hand in life: I have Friedreich's Ataxia and Scoliosis. Before you Google my disorders, let me explain. Friedreich's Ataxia is a progressive genetic nerve disorder that affects balance. Scoliosis is simply the curvature of the spine. So what? Everybody has something. My goal is to glean humour and happiness from adversity and hopefully to bring smiles to the faces of the people I meet along the road of life.

*****

So here I sit in the gymnasium, in October of 2010, about to graduate from Brock University with a degree in psychology. The speakers are going on and on. I can't doze off like someone sitting near the back of the audience. The graduation organizers put me in the front row for ease of access and so I could see the stage.

My parents, James and Rose McIntyre, are a few rows back over my left shoulder. Beside them sat my brother Will, his wife Julie, my brother Chad and his wife Nicole. The whole event was similar to a wedding, only it wasn't.

I wouldn't be where I am today without my family's ability to rally around me. We are a determined bunch. My family members enrich my life simply by being around me. If there is an activity that I wish to do, my family does their best to make it happen.

I know that there is emotion in the air. Every time I turn toward my family, I well up with tears. I can sense the pride in their eyes. If there were shirts with 'Team Meg' written on the front, they would all be happily wearing them. For now the shirts remain in my head.

I let my mind wander to the web of activities I've done that I didn't anticipate to be possible, while keeping a smile plastered on my face.

*****

In May of 1998, my best friend, Olivia Mason and I bought tickets to see the musical group the Backstreet Boys perform in Toronto. We both turn sixteen during the year. Olivia grew concerned that I would be able to go because I had scoliosis surgery scheduled in June. Fear of my coming procedure overtook my head space, but hope began to creep into my brain.

I had almost three months from my surgery to the date of the concert. If I couldn't go because I was bound to a bed in a hospital, I'd give my ticket to Olivia's sister Kate. The Make a Wish Foundation could surely pull some strings and get the Backstreet Boys to belt out some ballads at my bedside. But I digress…

The surgery date came up rather fast. I was as prepared as I could be. The pediatric orthopedic surgeon, Dr. Eduardo, would open up my back and insert two titanium rods and fuse them to my spine. Eventually my spine would grow around the rods.

Talking about the surgery left me naked and exposed to the world. At least I had an extra long summer and I didn't have to work at a part time job like most kids my age. Surgery wasn't a positive thought, but I was determined to look for the good in every situation.

August 22nd, 1998 arrived and I felt well enough to go to see the Backstreet Boys live. Let's be honest; I was going to the concert on a stretcher if I had to.

My conditions qualified me for Make a Wish, but I didn't care for other kids knowing my specific ailments. I preferred to let people see what is right with me. Nobody going through adolescence intended for other people to know details of personal medical history.

Chad thought I was a big nerd for going to a Backstreet Boys concert. Guys didn't appreciate the power a good boy band held over adolescent girls.

My parents drove us to the outdoor amphitheatre where the performance was held. My Dad wanted to put some music on in the minivan. That made me nervous because his taste in music wasn't the same as mine. When Neil Diamond's voice belted out some tunes over the speakers, I was slightly mortified.

After laughing hysterically at my Dad's choice of music, Olivia and I began to like Neil. Don't tell my Dad. Somebody call the nerd police.

My parents stopped in front of a distinct planter filled with purple petunias. We decided to meet there after the concert. Olivia and I joined the line to file onto the lawn… and what a lawn it was. The patchy grass was covered in goose shit. How on earth did they expect us to find a space to sit? I stared at the ground, searching for an area vacant of poop. While I fumed, Olivia found a spot clear of excrement.

We sat amongst hoards of hormonal teenage girls. A mixture of hairspray and Gap Dream perfumed the air around us. Any female with boobs had their girls on display for all to see. Ew. The whole venue reeked of desperation amongst the crowd of concert goers.

The frolicking females were foaming at the mouth like a group of rabid dogs. The anticipation of breathing the same air as the Boys was palpable. I'm sure I'm not the only one who has lain in bed at night wondering what it'd be like to lock lips with a Backstreet Boy.

The groups of girls standing behind us weren't people I wanted to get to know. They were talking about my scar that could be seen from the top of my black and white striped tank top. One of the girls suggested that I might be anorexic. I weighed ninety pounds, but I ate as much as a senior football player and that's not an exaggeration. Due to my disorder, I used up more energy than the average girl my age would necessitate in order to partake in daily life. I'm sure that my nerves ate up a bunch of calories just to walk down the school hall at dismissal time.

I stared at Olivia, hoping to snap out of a bad dream. My eyes were wet with tears that began to fall in slow motion. At that moment I knew I had a choice; leave now and always bow to the ways of inconsiderate people, or rise above petty things in search of my new normal. I chose to ignore their attempt at bullying and celebrated my life that day.

The crowd erupted in a loud scream as the Backstreet Boys made their way to the stage and began to sing. The main event had finally arrived.

After the concert ended we found my parents amongst the crowd. I leaned on my father for a moment. I had a raspy voice from screaming all afternoon and Olivia's hearing was never going to be the same. We began to move with the thousands of other people trying to remember where they parked their vehicles. I took my father's hand and looked up at him in silence.

Attending a concert was a good test of my stamina. My body utterly exhausted, I made my way back to the van. High school resumed in a few weeks and by then I planned to attend school full-time.

Being home schooled never hit my radar. My parents believed the social part of school to be an important part of a student's education and I wholeheartedly agreed with them. I had to resume my place on the imaginary social ladder.

After my recovery, I started to babysit again. I picked up with one family and gradually eased my way back into minding kids for most of the families I worked for before my surgery. I didn't babysit for the money. I couldn't believe the parents paid me to have fun with their children. Most of the people I babysat for were friends of my parents.

The Naughton and Wakowski families were friends that I babysat for at different times. Shortly after I had decided to return to babysitting, I was on a stool at the breakfast bar reading to the youngest Naughton children, her parents were almost ready to go out. A knock at the side door came and in walks Mr. Wakowski pointing his finger at the Naughton's who looked sheepishly back at him. The Naughton's had told the Wakowski's that my energy level was depleted and not ready to babysit, so I'd sit without any competition. I thought the whole situation to be rather funny. Apparently, I was hot commodity and didn't even realize it at the time.

I truly loved the families I babysat for. I made sure that each child had a chance to choose the board game or story. I often burned the popcorn, but the kids were well looked after while their parents went out. I babysat because I adored children. Kelsey Naughton told me her parents were keen on me coming over because I rounded up all of the sippy cups and spare plates and washed the dishes.

*****

The calendar sped forward to June of 1999 and I continued to fight for a new normal by landing my first summer job. Nepotism played a role thanks to my mother's friend. My duties entailed working at several information booths within Niagara Parks. My geography skills weren't exactly brilliant, but soon I learned how to give directions on an upside down map so the tourists could follow my advice.

Maybe someday I'd be able to laugh at the comical nature of my first day of work, but not as I slipped into the front seat of our dark green minivan. I was so tired and hungry. My mom went through a fast food drive-thru on our way home. As I sipped on a milkshake and nibbled on some French fries, I slowly came to life again.

We sold ticket packages to the attractions within Niagara Parks. I perused the different brochures when we weren't busy and raised any questions with my boss Melanie. While she had her lunch break, I was by myself in the information booth. I told a guy who had to go to Niagara-on-the-Lake that he had to go right instead of left on the Parkway, essentially sending him south to Fort Erie. I'm pretty sure he didn't believe me. If he followed the street signs he'd have gone north to his destination without a problem, but that wasn't exactly my best moment.

I liked interacting with the general public but on some days the tourists were lacking in intelligence. I wondered what those people did for a living in order to afford a vacation. Some of the minions had children with them. I wondered at the time about their sex lives… What the heck? Great. Now as I write I can't get the pictures out of my mind. How did we get into that position? No pun intended.

Now that I've led you to sex I may as well discuss my own sex life. I'm a virgin. There, my secret's out, floating in the air all around me. Of course I've thought about having my way with one of the Backstreet Boys. Or all of them? What teenage girl hasn't had those thoughts? Maybe Make a Wish could arrange that… A girl can dream.

Humans are funny creatures. There were moments I wanted to yell that I am normal and I possess the same thoughts and urges as other teenagers with raging hormones. I'll delve into my sexual side later, but the one man I was prepared to be with in every sense of the word turned out to be gay. God has a funny way of answering my prayers. Tiny boobs and a gay boyfriend weren't fulfilling my aspirations. When the time comes, God has some explaining to do.

Do I believe in God? Yes… no… kind of. I believe in a higher power watching over us. Sure, I lack answers to questions, but don't we all? Why did God choose me to suffer from a neurological disorder? I think He (or She), only gives a person what they can handle. God gave me to a family that is nothing short of amazing.

Without negativity, would we ever truly know what happiness is? If God isn't real, is it simply bad luck that dealt me a crappy hand at the poker table of life? Sure, life can be tough for anyone regardless of what abilities the person maintains. Life should be about the journey, not the destination. I'm not going to let a bad hand ruin my life. I believe I can rework how I play the cards, so that they work for me rather than against me.

The reason I brought up my first job was because it was a milestone for me. When I wasn't busy at work my boss was preparing wedding invitations for her sister's upcoming nuptials. Chatting about weddings forced me to think about the future and I wasn't sure I'd get married.

I hoped to have a boyfriend, an engagement, a wedding, a marriage, a home, a family, and a puppy. I may as well have a white picket fence surrounding my beautifully landscaped yard. I planned on having my Dad walk (or roll) me down the proverbial aisle. Dancing on my wedding day has been a dream since I was a wee girl. I pray that some of my dreams come true. DAMMIT.

Right now I'd go for a hug and kiss from someone of the male persuasion. There are women in courtships who receive more action than me and most of those couples don't allow a full frontal hug or a peck on the cheek before marriage. I'm not asking for the sun, moon, and stars.

At the end of the day I still have F. A., but I've never been a fan of labels. I can think for myself; I can talk and move my arms and legs. My mind is intact. There are hobbies I can do that make what I can't do seem relatively minor. I learned to ride a bike before my disorder took hold. I played baseball and hide and seek with the neighbourhood kids.

For fun I liked to read, write and watch movies. If my mood was full of extra patience, I'd attempt to make friendship bracelets. I could do most activities; I just had to have a plan of attack.

A few months after I turned sixteen I studied the driver's manual until I couldn't see anything but the answers floating in my mind. One of my doctors referred to driving and I just wasn't ready to learn to drive. He didn't say I couldn't or shouldn't drive. I was afraid to bring it up with anyone, for fear they'd shut me down.

One day I woke up and I knew I had prepared enough to take the written driving test. I crossed my fingers and toes at that moment in time, hoping I would receive my beginner's driving license. I was the only person taking the test that day, so I had my choice of seat. The front row was lonely, but I managed to pass the test with flying colours.

Days after I had my beginning license, my mother brought me to deserted park off the beaten path to practice my driving skills. Well, by the time we switched drivers, I was in a right knot.

Even though the spring air was breezy, I was sweaty. My short sleeve plaid shirt was starting to show the sweat under my arms. Damn light coloured shirts. I put my hands at 10 and 2, adjusted my seat to where it felt comfortable. I took a deep breath and put the car in gear.

I thought that once I got going my mood would calm down. This didn't happen. I was worried that if I was this anxious about driving with my mother, how would I manage when I had a van full of teenagers.

A couple days passed and my Mom and I went to a mall parking lot after the shoppers and employees had left for home, to try driving once more. I didn't know it then, but having wide open spaces all around me didn't help. I couldn't determine a reference point. The building was built on a slight angle to the curbing.

The parking lines were faded from years of wear, so I couldn't find my balance in the van. At the time, I had trouble vocalizing what my internal thoughts were saying. I reminded myself I differed from most people. If everybody came out the same, the world wouldn't be interesting.

Both times I got behind the wheel of our minivan I was alarmed at the size of the vehicle. I didn't know if I would be capable of driving alone or with other people regardless of the rider's age. The thought of being responsible for the van terrified me. My confidence was hindered by a degenerative neuromuscular condition. I might be better suited to being a passenger.

*****

By the time October of 2004 rolled around, I battled my body's gradual decline. Sometimes reality bites. I often wondered whether I'd be attractive to any man because I used a wheelchair. There would be advantages though, like rolling away from a boring conversation. If I had a fight with my husband, I could run over his toes. If stubbing your toe was any indication, it wouldn't be pretty.

My mind was rampant with emotional pain. My body ached with longing to be like other young adults. I remember the setting autumn sun streaming in through the kitchen window, as I watched my Mom peel apples for dessert that evening. I wondered what she was thinking behind her honey coloured eyes. There was silence and yet the secret bond between mother and daughter was in every breath we took.

My Mom wanted me to be more at peace with my place in the world. Inside my heart I knew it was time I started using a wheelchair when I left the house. With no assistance, I found staying upright to be shaky at best. My balance remained steady at next to nil. I wasn't able to have fun when I did go out because I was too busy trying not to fall flat on my face.

To be seen as different from anybody else was never a goal. I couldn't just sit there and let my body deteriorate. I had people to see, places to go, and things to do. Thinking about the future made me fearful… Under my circumstances, control over my physical being was slipping through my hands like a smooth silk shirt.

I worried people I grew up with would view me differently if they saw me in a wheelchair. There's the old saying that people who mind don't matter and those who matter don't mind. That was true, but I just couldn't apply this to my own situation.

*****

The glass paneled front door swung open and in walked my older brother Chad and his wife Nicole. Chad always made my day better. His smile was calming.

We were having apple crisp that night and there was beef stew in the slow cooker that would be ready for dinner. Chad could smell an apple crisp over the phone.

Chad and Nicole invited me to go to the mall with them. I decided to go with them because I rarely miss a shopping opportunity. Soon after, Nicole asked my brother to get our Great Aunt's old wheelchair from the garage. How could I back out of this now? They tricked me into going to the mall with them.

My Aunt Beatrice had been in her nineties when she began having issues with her mobility. For her, using a wheelchair was age related degeneration. She's been gone for quite some time now. At that point, I wondered what sitting my ass in an ancient wheelchair would be like. I don't think I could handle if the chair smelled of moth balls. What if there were indentations in the cushion from the previous owner?

My mother told me it'd be fine and I knew she was probably right, but I couldn't ignore the uneasiness in the pit of my stomach.

The shopping voyage went better than I expected. Nobody gave me a second look while I was in the wheelchair. We didn't see anyone that any of us knew. I was scared of that. My school friends had seen me walk. People asking questions or gossiping about the condition I was in, was something I could do without.

Nicole coaxed me to look into getting my own custom wheelchair. She was right. I had to investigate and find out what was involved in getting my own wheelchair. My Aunt Beatrice's chair was alright for now, but after a while my ass went numb. In order to gather information about assistive devices I had to email someone at a store that supplied and sold medical aids to the public.

Dear Shopper's Home Healthcare,
I'm a 22 year old with Friedreich's Ataxia and think it is time to have my own manual wheelchair.
How do I go about doing so?
Megan McIntyre

I guess that the staff at Shopper's Home Healthcare had jobs before I wrote to the company, so I shouldn't have hovered over my computer waiting for an answer to my email. A few hours later I heard the familiar ping that indicated new mail had arrived.

Dear Megan,
I'd be happy to meet with you in person to go over all of the options for your new wheelchair.
I'll set you up with several wheelchairs to try, so you can find out what works for you and what doesn't. It's a similar process to buying a car.
Have a look at www.invacare.com and tell me what you like. I'll work on getting some wheelchairs to test drive. I'll set up an appointment with an Occupational Therapist to size and fit the wheelchair once we have an idea what make and model you need.
I know the process may seem overwhelming at first. Through a process of elimination, we will find you the right match.
Noelle Raven

Shopper's Home Healthcare sent Noelle to my house the next week. The whole process of getting a chair took six months. Because I had never had a wheelchair before, it took longer to zero in on what type of chair worked for me. Noelle brought a sample folding chair with her for me to try for a month.

I browsed the website Noelle suggested and several other sites I'd come across. As long as the chair I ended up with didn't have the name 'Quickie 2' written on my rear, I'd be alright. It was bad enough that I'd never had sex; I shouldn't be reminded of what I was missing out on every day. That being said, the names of the wheelchairs had hilarious connotations. I couldn't use a chair that said 'Sunshine Quickie' across my backside. I wished I was joking.

It took some encouragement, but I now had a wheelchair and the world seemed doable. Nicole showed me that using a wheelchair wasn't the end of the world, but rather a fresh start.

February of 2004 had begun and winter had left mountains of snow. My new wheelchair was delivered and I couldn't wait to break it in. My Dad agreed to take me to the big box plaza after dinner one night.

I was terrified we'd see someone I knew. My Dad tried to ease my worries. His plan was to keep right on trucking, which didn't do much for my anxiety.

I sighed and swung my tiny bum into my glossy black wheelchair and we entered the store. Our neighbours, the Alison's came over and spoke to us briefly. They didn't say a peep about my wheelchair. Perhaps my Dad was right: I worried too much. Let's keep this between us.

I see now, everyone wasn't my enemy. Of course some people would stop and look me over. Sometimes a person was uncomfortable around me due to a lack of experience with disabled people. When I started to speak, the average person didn't know how to respond. If a human being is truly ignorant, I have no trouble talking and breaking the preconceived notion that someone in a wheelchair must not be able to speak or is lacking in intellect. Everyone is different; we didn't all wear the same sized shoe or learn to ride a bike at the same moment.

*****

I closed my eyes for what seemed like a second and five years went by. My brother Will was talking about going to the gun range for target shooting. He offered to take anybody who wanted to go with him.

He'd taken his wife Julie and she got joy out of aiming and shooting at a target. I offered to go, if it was possible for somebody in a wheelchair to shoot at a target. Will didn't know either, but he'd check it out with the gun range and get back to me.

Will said I could go to the gun range with him and his hunting buddy Lenny Tomlins. My Dad wondered how that would work with my bad shoulder. I thought about that. When I pictured myself shooting a gun, it's always left handed. Will and Lenny are both left handed so I figured they'd show me how to prepare to shoot.

My Dad wanted to know about the kick back from the gun. William decided to teach me to shoot on a 22 caliber rifle which had no kick back. I knew my parents were unsure about sending their daughter to a gun range, but Will was ultra safety conscious. I'd never met Lenny before we went to the range, but I was sure nobody would mess with me when I was with two muscular guys. My parents trusted Will; it's the unpredictable nature of other people and guns that made them anxious. Accidents happened and fathers wouldn't stop worrying about their daughters.

Once we had the targets set up on the range, Will instructed me to always treat a gun as if it's loaded. Once I was comfortable I took the safety off. I could see the target in the crosshairs and I was ready to fire.

My ear protection was on. I took the shot. Looking down the field with binoculars, I could see that I hit the target. My lips curved upwards into a toothy grin. I didn't care that the bullet hole wasn't dead centre. I was hooked and wanted to do take another shot. Will and Lenny cheered. Firing a gun at a target was an incredible stress relief. Who knew? I had completed an item on my bucket list.

I had a sudden surge of energy. I was a decent shot. My disability didn't make my learning to shoot any harder. In fact, because I was so aware of the linear spaces around me, lining up my shot was easier than I had thought. I noticed that when adult males walked by, they paused to watch a first time shooter bask in the glory of their accomplishments. My bright fuchsia jacket may have screamed that I was new to the gun range; my smile showed the onlookers that I'd be back. I was serious about refusing to let other people set limitations for me.

On the way home, I felt closer to Will. I learned about the hobby that he took part in. There would always be an age gap between Will and me, but we found time for each other to further cement our relationship.

Wheelchairs are not the barrier to life that I thought they were. I learned that a wheelchair is an assistive device that helps me to see the planet from a new perspective. I had to maintain a positive attitude. The alternative wasn't pretty.

*****

"Looks like we made it, we might've taken the long way, but it looks like we made it after all." I hummed the Shania Twain song to myself as I faced the stage.

Macaroni & Alphabet Soup

When are they going to stop the rambling speeches and hand out our degrees? Some people who got a hold of a microphone didn't know when to let it go. I began to daydream, with a half-smile appropriately gracing my face as the convocation ceremony continued.

*****

At thirteen years of age, I was about to enter high school. A scary thought for an average teenager, but I was far from your standard adolescent. I'm sure every girl in school had bigger boobs than I did and that wasn't hard because I only weighed seventy-two pounds.

My Mom told me nobody is perfect. Some people pay big bucks for the shiny blonde hair I come by naturally. Everyone has an issue of some sort: some are external fights and others have internal struggles. I sat staring at the sea of students dressed head to toe in preppy clothes with brand names in large lettering. My brothers had finished high school, but I wanted both of them to magically appear so I didn't have to be alone on my brief walk into high school.

My Mom reminded me that we would see the doctor in a few days to discuss my troubles. Maybe I was just a late bloomer like she had been. I had better get a move on, or I'd be late for my first day. My Mom was careful about her words and actions so she wouldn't appear visibly bothered.

I slammed the door of my mother's car and walked up the path to the entrance of the school, tripping on the small step as I reached for the door. At least I didn't fall. The doors were super heavy and my petite frame made it harder to open the door. Maybe I would have to use the button to automatically open the door, but I wanted to be like everyone else.

I wasn't angry at my mother, although it did appear that way. My life circumstances weren't what I wished for. I hoped to learn to be more even tempered.

When I registered for high school the human resources staff assigned each student a locker. As I placed my combination lock on the door of my locker, I realized that my small self would likely fit inside the tiny space. I didn't aim to have anyone test my theory out. I was anxious to see what my first day would be like. On top of first day jitters, I was getting angry that puberty had left me in the dark.

I saw Ava Hollingsworth, a friend from my elementary school. I was so happy to find a familiar face among all of the strangers. High school was so much bigger than our former school.

A really attractive guy came up near me and I was at a loss for words. As he put his backpack in the locker two over from mine, I smiled. He said his name was Caleb Finnegan, but his friends referred to him as Finn. I remained silent until I remembered my own name. His sister and I shared the same name. I hit the jackpot as far as locker buddies go. Caleb smelled of men's deodorant with a touch of woodsy musk that I presumed was his cologne.

*****

The next afternoon, I was on my way to the office of my family doctor with my mother. I had to talk about my constant struggle to gain weight. I know that being underweight didn't seem like a horrible problem to have, but I had just started the ninth grade and hadn't yet had a regular period. I felt something was amiss, but I couldn't put my finger on it.

Dr. Miles Thatcher was my Grandma Porter's family doctor too, so he was aware that we didn't come running to him for every ache and pain. He was the ideal family physician; he always knew what to do or who to ask. My parents were grateful he took our family on when our former doctor retired. Dr. Thatcher had four girls of his own; my mother assured me he would treat me as if I was one of his own children.

As I was sitting on the examination table, I wondered if my concerns were valid. Had I become impatient in my wait for puberty to begin? Was I normal? If only I knew that I wasn't the only teenager that questioned whether they fit in with other high school students.

Everything looked to be in order, but the doctor would like to send me to a pediatrician, to look a few things over. Dr. Apollo would look over my development to see if anything was out of place.

A week later my Mom and I sat in the pediatricians' waiting room. What was next? I tried to distract myself with a magazine, but I noticed it was from January 1993, and so I decided to pass on fashion updates that were nearly a decade old.

Dr. Eve Apollo entered the exam room; her melodic European accent filled the sterile surroundings. She noticed that I was underweight. She had a motherly vibe about her and I liked her as soon as she entered the exam room.

Dr. Apollo wanted to know if I was afraid of the dark. I should hope not, I was thirteen years old. My milky skin became a dark hue of pink and my mother looked intrigued by the doctor's line of questioning.

The doctor wondered if I walked to the bathroom in the night with no lights on. What a specific question. I wondered what she was getting at.

I thought about the other day when I went to a school dance. The gym was dark and dry ice flowed around people's feet. I had trouble navigating, but so did a lot of kids.

I don't usually have to use the bathroom in the night, but if I do, I turn on my reading lamp. I can be klutzy at the best of times, but I think the darkness accentuates my lack of coordination. Isn't everybody like that? I was lost in thought.

It might have been nothing. Teenagers are still getting used to their growing bodies and that can make for an uncoordinated state. Dr. Apollo said we'd get to the bottom of this together. Her soothing voice was of some comfort to me.

The doctor noticed a few puzzling issues during my examination. She noticed that when I closed my eyes, my body swayed back and forth. Dr. Apollo referred me to a neurologist for further testing. She noticed a curvature of my spine and made a referral for me to see an orthopedic surgeon.

*****

One day I called Ava after school to discuss the welcome back to school dance that happened week before. A slow dance had come over the speakers, so I backed up to sit on the sidelines with some friends. Caleb proposed we dance and I confessed I looked over my shoulder to see if a pretty girl was behind me. He took my hand and led me to the dance floor. I took a deep breath in and reveled in the smell of his body spray, trying not to step on his feet. When the dance ended, I reluctantly stepped out of the safety his arms and Caleb told me he'd see me at school.

Caleb and I flirted with each other by the lockers. The school board decided high school freshmen should be with the same students all day, so they could find their way together. I felt comfortable walking to class with Caleb.

*****

By the middle of October I still didn't know why I came home exhausted at the end of each day. A little sleepiness is expected during adolescence, but I had a three hour nap after school, just to get by. My brothers noticed my sleepy state and they each led busy lives.

My parents and I showed up at the Children's Hospital to see Dr. O'Connor, the pediatric neurologist who had been recommended. A doctor doesn't send you to a hospital for a hang nail. If my doctors sent me to a specialist, I trusted their reasoning. What it was, I didn't know.

The hallway was colourful and had an "Under the Sea" theme, but the examining room was devoid of colour. The only sign of life was the lone orange crayon on the low table in the corner.

Several minutes went by and the door opened. Dr. Tabitha O'Connor wouldn't shake my hand. She ignored me. She didn't look any of us in the eye.

"I don't like teenagers and they don't like me." The doctor's words didn't inspire confidence in her. When you have the personality of a doorknob, you can't expect people to connect with you on any level.

Dr. O'Connor directed me to perform a few neurological tests. She wanted me to stand up and close my eyes. I did as directed; I wobbled and may have fallen if I hadn't opened my eyes. She stood behind me in case I fell, but I didn't trust her one bit.

Dr. O'Connor had me follow her finger with my eyes. Next, I was to touch my nose with one finger and then touch her finger. I considered picking my nose and wiping a booger on her hand, but I refrained. My parents smiled at me when I completed the tasks, even though they saw my accuracy wasn't a hundred percent.

The doctor had to do a blood test to confirm what she thought might be going on. A nurse came in to draw a vial of my blood. Her scrubs seemed to be new. She was obviously fresh from university. I endured four separate pin pricks to get blood. My Mom begged me to keep my body hydrated. The lack of fluids made my veins hard to find for even the most experienced technician.

I believed Doctor O'Connor was a bitch. I slipped off of the chair and leaned on my Dad before continuing to walk to the reception desk. Normally my mother would argue, but she couldn't say I was wrong.

The wavy design in the carpet made me somewhat dizzy. Luckily I could follow a railing with my eyes. I wondered if everybody did that…

We made a follow-up appointment in eight weeks time with the receptionist and made our way to the elevators. My parents and I were not impressed with Dr. O'Connor's sociability.

The eight weeks were stressful for the whole family. Nobody could control the outcome of the blood test and that frightened all of us.

Chad used laughter to perk everyone up. He would sing, "Caleb and Megan sitting in a tree". I would giggle along as he sang, trying to not to laugh but failing.

Will talked in a soft, soothing voice. He wrapped his arms around me frequently and kissed the top of my head.

Will taught me how to burp the alphabet as a distraction. When my brothers attended high school, a burping contest was held during lunchtime and a girl won. Will and Chad wanted me to be prepared to win, if the occasion should arise. Much to my parents' dismay, I was quite proficient at burping. They taught my brothers and me not to belch in front of our grandmothers. We had to know our audience.

*****

No matter what the test results showed, my family would figure out a way to make life work. Together we formed a strong family unit.

My parents tried to keep our schedules as normal as possible, but I knew they were worried. There was something about the way my parents looked at each other when they were sipping their morning cup of coffee that let me know they were upset. I wasn't sure what I was feeling.

When Will was six years old he had to have several brain surgeries. He had inflammation of the brain and at the time, the outcome didn't look good. My parents experienced the anxiety of having a sick child. Will was a fighter. I learned how to be tough from my big brothers.

November came and went; I should have been in a happy mood because my birthday was just around the bend. Instead I was riding in the elevator up to Dr. O'Connor's clinic with my parents.

I didn't like her. I prayed for a miracle. She was awful at relating to people. My parents found her mannerisms to be strange and unprofessional. If we could get through this appointment, we'd see what our options were.

I expected there might be another pediatric neurologist in the children's hospital.

Dr. O'Connor came out to the waiting room and greeted us with a severe nod. When I stood up to follow her, she asked me to wait there while she talked to my parents.

My parents disappeared into an office behind the doctor and I was all by myself in the waiting room with nothing but my thoughts to keep me company.

What a bitch the doctor was being. I mean she must have known that we had all worried ourselves sick and she chose to leave me out of my appointment. I wasn't four years old. I was fourteen... Dammit.

Here's the thoughts I remembered cycling through my head at the time. What the hell was wrong with me? Is my diagnosis so bad that the doctor had to tell my parents first? Did I have cancer? Is chemo going to be part of my treatment? Is my hair going to fall out? Not my hair, oh please no. Am I going to die soon? Or did I have some rare disease that nobody had ever heard of? I just wanted to be normal. What is normal anyway? Did I have multiple sclerosis? Would a wheelchair be in my future? Oh fudge.

The nurse came and got me and I followed her into the room where my parents had been chatting with the doctor. I sat in an empty chair next to my Dad and an eerie chill went through my body. I grabbed a hold of my father's hand. I was scared and putting my hand in his was soothing to me.

Dr. O'Connor told me I had Friedreich's Ataxia, a degenerative nerve disorder that has no cure. F.A. was genetic in nature and affects a person's balance. My unsteadiness began to make sense. She spoke in a monotone voice and no emotion whatsoever.

I'd never be a tight rope walker or a high wire acrobat. I giggled at the thought. I had never even dreamed of doing those things. I wanted bigger boobs, not a major disease. I must speak to God; He got the answer to my prayers all wrong.

Dr. O'Connor offered to give us the name of a boy who also had Friedreich's Ataxia. She said his family was nerdy just like us. Because we used computers, she labeled us as nerds? Dr. O'Connor had no bedside manner. I didn't pursue meeting anyone she suggested.

Calling a young teenage girl nerdy didn't go over well with my parents. Only Chad calls me a nerd because it's a term of endearment between us.

If Will and Chad had been at the appointment, they would have risen off the chairs to defend me. Nobody was ever going to hurt their little sister, physically or emotionally. Whenever I got down on myself, my family pulled me out of my funky mood.

Meeting someone else with my disorder ranked rather low on my to-do-list. I had no intentions of seeing someone better off than me because I'd feel negatively about myself. Someone worse off than me wouldn't be a good situation because I'd be waiting for the poor mobility to come. I just got my diagnosis and my family should take some time to understand the disorder before I went and made friends. A friendship based on two people having the same disability seemed artificial and not my style. Can you say awkward?

I resolved to not live under a label. My conversations wouldn't open a discussion of my disability. I was a person before I was diagnosed and I would continue to be a person afterwards. I'm Megan first and foremost. I was happy to talk, just not a disability centered conversation.

Some people dwell on the negative parts of their lives. I couldn't figure out why a segment of the disabled population had to tell you a small dose of their ailment within thirty seconds of encountering them.

Dr. O'Connor had accepted a job in Halifax, so my next appointment would be with a new doctor. The receptionist had the details and would coordinate my next visit. Somebody listened to my thoughts. Halifax was far enough away for the bitch to go. Tokyo would have been better, but beggars can't be choosers. Sometimes things have a way of working out.

The bitch was finally gone. Someone kept an eye on my family from heaven above. I had some answers and while my diagnosis wasn't fabulous news, the waiting game had finished. We started to get a handle on the disorder I faced. I couldn't wipe the grin off my face because Dr. O'Connor left my life for good. Surely in a research position, she wouldn't have to interact with people very often.

*****

Happy New Year. My parents and I were headed to the children's hospital for yet another appointment. I was seeing a pediatric orthopedic surgeon about my curved spine. First I had a standing back x-ray done, so the doctor could examine the films before I saw him.

Dr. Quinn Eduardo was my orthopedic surgeon. He looked through Gucci glasses at me and smiled. His warm demeanor made me relax instantly.

My spine had a slight curvature that could be seen on the x-rays.

The doctor said I had scoliosis, or an abnormal curvature of the spine. Scoliosis sounded like the name of a horror movie.

The doctor arranged for a mould of my torso to be made. From the mould, a back brace would be formed. The doctor hoped the brace would prevent or slow the progression of the curvature. If the brace didn't help, surgical methods would be used to straighten my spine.

My head filled with new terms. The idea of wearing a back brace in high school didn't sound like fun at all. I snapped out of my fog in time to hear the doctor say that the brace would be worn at night only.

I get to pick the colour and pattern of the brace though. My eyes were alight with wonder. I'd wear pyjamas in the day if flannel was acceptable attire. Since my back brace would essentially be my new night wear, it had to be flashy. If the firemen had to carry me out of my house like a princess; I had to look just right. I fantasized for a brief moment.

Dr. Eduardo laughed as he rested his hand on my shoulder with a twinkle in his dark brown eyes. He looked as though he'd been listening to my inner chatter. I didn't mind. In fact, it bonded us.

The hospital had a family information center that Dr. Eduardo wanted us to visit on our way out. The doctor motioned toward the door and ushered us out of the exam room. Dr. Eduardo saw the worry in my Dad's face while he blotted a teardrop from his own sun kissed wrinkled cheek on a tissue. My Dad shook his hand and I knew everything would turn out just fine.

Hannah Green was the kinesiology student on duty in the information room. She did a few searches on a medical search engine and printed off a few articles for us to take home and digest. Hannah told us not to search the internet about my disorders. A lot of false medical information lay in the weeds of the internet. Nobody needed to fret about false data.

The gray sky seeped in through the windows of the hospital courtyard. Seriously? I had faith the weather wasn't a metaphor for what the future would be like. A tiny ray of sunshine poked through the clouds, which made me smile.

In order to make a mould of my back I had to visit the orthopedic hospital. The technicians prepared what looked like a giant bowl of runny oatmeal and a stack of enormous sterile strips. Next, they began a process that resembled paper-mâché. I had to lie without much movement. Since my boobs were nothing more than ant hills, I had a perfect view of the goings on around me.

When I became nervous I couldn't pee. I was thankful for that. The clinicians hurried to complete the mould of my torso before the goo hardened like cement. I did notice a tightening of the fibers as the liquid dried up.

The temperature beneath the shell became quite warm. In fact, I even broke a sweat. I suffered the heat in June and September while I was in school. I preferred air conditioning whenever possible.

The winter progressed at a snail's pace. We headed to meet Dr. O'Connor's replacement. Anybody else would be an improvement. I glanced out the back seat of the van in time to see snow falling ever so slowly. The ground sparkled after the snowfall.

My parents and I sat in the waiting room of my new neurologist. My new doctor's name was Dr. R. Nasty. I questioned what the R stood for. Perhaps his first name was Ray or Ross. Or maybe it stood for Really.

Dr. Rowan Nasty was a new pediatric neurologist at the McMaster Children's Hospital. I didn't know it at the time, but I was one of Dr. Nasty's first patients as a full-fledged pediatric neurologist. He put his hand out to shake my hand and I was reassured by his calming presence. This doctor was definitely not nasty in anyway. I had faith in his abilities. As long as I was under Dr. Nasty's care, my world would be better because of him.

He stood before me, a gorgeous specimen flashing his dimples. With my permission, Dr. Nasty started some neurological tests, not the kind of tests you have in school.

I stared up at the doctor, who dressed in khaki pants and a blue dress shirt. He looked like he had been ripped from a Gap ad, with his short dark hair and cleanly shaven face. He grinned, not wanting to squash my cheerful spirit.

I truly loved Dr. Nasty, not in a romantic sense. He piloted my medical ship and I trusted him with my life. Of course, it didn't hurt that he was good looking. When he walked in, I understood he was going to blow the previous bitch doctor out of the water.

Dr. Nasty should be called Dr. Eye Candy. His model appearance would definitely be a hit with the mothers of his patients. I don't know where he came from or why he chose to land at the hospital I went to, but whatever the reason, I was forever grateful.

Dr. Nasty had brawn and brains, what's not to like? He had a fabulous manner with me and my parents. I'm sure Dr. Nasty treated all his patients the same way, but I felt special. Having a doctor that took the time to explain the terms in plain English made the journey a little less overwhelming.

We went off to the heart lab, down the hall in the yellow section of the hospital. People with Friedreich's Ataxia should be seen by a cardiologist regularly to monitor overall heart health.

I wasn't sure what an echocardiogram entailed, but I soon found out. Once I settled on a hospital bed, the technician began. An echocardiogram is basically an ultrasound of the heart. A wand, not unlike a computer mouse was used to look at the heart. The clinician smeared cold jelly on it, rubbed the wand over my chest and the heart appeared on the monitor. When I was finished having my heart test, the images were sent to the cardiologist for close examination.

The following month I saw Dr. Savannah Branch, a cardiologist at the McMaster Children's Hospital. I wasn't anxious about coming to the hospital anymore. I liked the atmosphere there. Everyone I met was friendly and the staff seemed to genuinely like their jobs.

The doctor told me that my heart looked good. Dr. Branch wanted to repeat the test and see me again in six months. She would monitor me closely to prevent any damage to the heart muscle. The doctor kept an eye on my heart. She didn't intend to wait until I had an issue and play the catch-up game.

Dr. Branch had the curly hair every straight haired girl dreamed of. I wanted long curly hair, good grades, an athletic body, a popular personality and a muscular boyfriend. High school and puberty were hard enough without a genetic disorder hanging over my head.

I supposed if I ended up needing to use a wheelchair, at least I'd be able to take advantage of the front row parking everywhere I went. There was a plus side to most activities; I just had to dig deep to find the upside.

*****

In May, the hospital telephoned to say my back brace was ready for pick up. My Mom and I arrived for my fitting the next afternoon. Secretly I had dreamed that the hospital would somehow lose my brace and I'd have to wait while they constructed a new one.

The brace definitely didn't provide any comfort. The hard plastic was unforgiving. When I put the brace on, I felt like I had a cast on my torso. My complaints were nearly enough for my mother to turn around and forget the brace altogether.

Summer came around and the heat had risen to near unbearable temperatures. Thank goodness for air conditioning. My mother liked the cold air to hit you in the face when you stepped into the house. The back brace was hot and sweat inducing, even with the air conditioning cranked down low.

Chad was concerned for my well-being. His bedroom shared a wall with mine, so he often heard me chuck the brace onto the floor or moan in pain. He didn't like to see me hurt and not know what to do to fix the issue.

Will's bedroom was downstairs and he would hear the Velcro being undone and finally the thud the brace made when the plastic hit the floor. He too wished that he could make my life better.

My family may not have realized it at the time, but each of them brought sunshine to my life on a cloudy day. My parents and brothers, along with my extended family and close friends, provided me with the strength and encouragement to continue moving forward, even when the pathway seemed to be littered with obstacles.

Chad would often lean in my bedroom doorway and say something goofy. Some people might have been irritated, but not me. I looked forward to his silly antics. In that moment, I focused on the humorous bits of life and every other thought fell to the floor.

I usually ripped the brace off in my sleep, even though the corset did me no good while on the floor. The alarm sounded for my parents when the Velcro ripped. My parents only wanted what the very best for me. When they spoke firmly to me, I came to the conclusion they lacked sleep. My parents wanted so badly to trade places with me, but that wasn't possible.

My mind told me I should wear the back brace, but none of us had had a good night's sleep in a long while. If the brace didn't hold my curved spine, surgery would be performed. Surgery always lingered at the back of my brain.

November came and I turned fifteen. Fall was nearly over and the days got shorter. My mood mirrored the dark and cloudy weather.

My mother checked me in to see Dr. Eduardo. She gave my health card to the receptionist behind the counter. The lady told my mother that I had touched Dr. Eduardo's heart in a way that nobody else had. My Mom blinked rapidly to try and keep the tears from falling down her face. My Mom joined my Dad and me in the seating area.

My Dad gazed at my mother with inquisitive eyes. As tears stung her eyes, dribbling down her cheeks, she began to explain. My cheerful personality brought out Dr. Eduardo's inner happiness. He smiled from ear to ear as I approached the clinic doorway.

A few minutes later Dr. Eduardo entered the room, showing off his white teeth. Based on my most recent x-rays, the brace wasn't holding my spinal curve as much as he'd expected it would.

Dr. Eduardo recommended I have an operation. Surgery? I didn't like the idea of an incision along the middle of my back. Two titanium rods placed along the length of my spine would straighten my spinal column. Surgery. Ahhh.

I would have a scar from the nape of my neck to just above my bum. My back pain might increase temporarily, in exchange for long term gain.

I may end up having some limitations, but the doctor suspected I'd find a way to do most activities. My stubborn determination was quite evident in our brief interactions.

The surgery wouldn't be a cake walk. My parents trusted Dr. Eduardo would prepare me for what happened before, during and after surgery.

February, 1998 approached and a foot of packing snow seemed to get deeper by the day. The ice patches on tne roads made for a slippery adventure. The snow hadn't yet turned to the brown slush, so the drifts still remained pure white.

On our way to see Dr. Eduardo, my emotions jumbled up. The best way to get a straight spine would be surgery. Dr. Eduardo wanted to do the surgery right away, but agreed to a date near the end of the school year. I could recuperate over the summer and not be worried over missing assignments.

What about my final marks? I disliked tests, but not many kids got excited over exams. My parents had an appointment with my guidance counsellor, Mr. Dillard to discuss what had to be done in terms of my finals.

My parents and guidance counsellor all agreed it would be better for me if I didn't write exams in June. My teachers would average my marks for the semester. I could tell my best friends Olivia Mason and Tyler Finlay, but not the whole school.

One stress I could do without leading up to surgery was exams. Not having to write my finals took a load off my mind. If I never conjugated a French verb ever again, it'd be too soon.

Time seemed to fly by. I blinked and May appeared. My pre-op day arrived and I hurried to get myself ready. My sandals tended to be difficult to put on. My flipping' Birkenstocks looked fabulous, but the buckles proved hard to do up. My fifteen year old self thought the brand provided relief to my aching feet.

The first stop, I needed blood work done. The lab was on the main floor in the yellow section of the hospital. On the way to the outpatient blood work area, we passed a sign that pointed to the Endoscopy Unit. Olivia's mother, Josie, worked in the endoscopy department at a hospital closer to home. The doctors stuck a fine camera up your bum to look for signs of infection or disease. A jackhammer could be heard coming from the hall. Someone got the shit pounded out of them in endoscopy. The laughter cut the tension.

Soon enough, we flipped the calendar over to June and my surgery date was on the second. I tried not to be scared shitless of surgery, but I failed. I'd go to sleep being five feet two inches and wake up being five feet six inches tall. Not bad for being asleep.

Will and Chad hugged me before I went to bed. Will kept his emotions in check, so that we wouldn't all fall apart into a tumble of tears. Will was great in times of high stress.

When I turned ten, Will bought me a 'lil' brother fishing rod. He taught me how to fish. We went out for dinner periodically and had long talks about the future.

Chad wore his feelings on his sleeve. His concern for my well-being caused his eyes to nearly overflow. He leaned in for one last hug. Chad grew terrified that he would never get to make me laugh again or call me a nerd. Whatever activity we took on, ended up being fun. Chad would go swimming with me and do crazy moves off of the diving board. Chad's animated expressions made me giggle until I hurt.

Dr. Eduardo went down the hall with his lunch pail in his hand. He was planning on being done my surgery by lunchtime. I wondered what kind of lunch he brought. My menu for today consisted of chicken broth and a side of ice-chips.

Dr. Eduardo and his team completed a successful six hour surgery.

My nurse wanted to know where my parents would be staying the night. They bunked at my Auntie Leona and Uncle Ted's home in Burlington. Neither one of my parents knew their phone number, but I did. Most of the time my head is filled with useless information. My groggy voice spit out the phone number slowly. I memorized the number long ago. I drifted back to sleep because my Mom nodded her head to the nurse.

Once I moved out of the pediatric intensive care unit onto the children's floor, my Mom stayed in the room with me.

Dr. Eduardo came through my room on his rounds. He scanned the room and looked at all the flowers, teddy bears, and cards. So many people cared for me and sent their love from far and wide. What a lucky girl to be among so much affection.

My Dad took a deep breath and peeked at my scar. He raised his hands in disbelief. The stitches lay in a straight line because a curved scar is less desirable.

My brother Will entered my hospital room and I gazed up at him through watery eyes. He and I embraced carefully, so as not to cause me any pain. At almost ten years older than me, the years faded fast. He handed me a bouquet of pink, red, and yellow roses.

Chad arrived a short time later. We hugged in silence. He sniffled and stared at me as tears dripped onto my shoulders. Chad may be not quite seven years older, but the age gap seemed to shrink as we grew up. He had a soft spot for me. He handed me a small teddy bear with a red heart on his sweater.

My best friend Olivia Mason, her sister Kate, Mom and Nan stopped by to check on my recovery. Olivia thought all hospitals smelled like hand sanitizer.

Liv and Kate's Grandpa wanted to send fresh strawberries to get me pooping again. Nobody received privacy in the hospital. I gave my Mother the stink eye for slightly longer than necessary.

Josie rubbed her hands together. Olivia turned away and everybody else caught a glimpse of my scar. "I'm impressed at how neat the incision turned out!" Josie admired the staples once more.

Blood made Olivia squeamish, so she continued to peer out my hospital room door. She sat facing the window while her family took in my bandaged back.

After a few days, I got to make some food choices for meals the following day. Even as a teenager, I liked having macaroni and cheese or alphabet soup. In fact, the menu brought me back to my own childhood and that made being in the hospital easier.

A volunteer tapped on my open door. After he stepped inside the door, he presented me a hand knitted blanket made by hospital volunteers. I managed to thank the man in the green vest. The chevron knitted blanket added colour to my bed.

I couldn't be released from the hospital until I went poo. The liquid laxative made me throw up. Perhaps, being scared shitless about surgery was a poor choice of words. What goes in must eventually come out. Right? The medicine tasted awful.

Chad left the room because seeing me upset got to him. A little fresh air and his rosy complexion returned.

I signaled to my Mother to move toward the restroom immediately. My Mom hurried me down the hall, the I.V. pole rolling between us. A while later we emerged with a smile gracing my Mom's petite mouth. The nurses behind the station looked at me expectantly. My mother said nothing, but raised two thumbs up as we moseyed back to my room. The nurses clapped their hands and cheered as I skulked down the hallway. Thank goodness my cell phone didn't include a video camera. I could have been in a viral video. The headline would read: Girl Shits and the Crowd Goes wild.' 'Pooper Parade. Plop, Plop, Hooray.

The hospital discharged me on my eighth day post-surgery. The summer heat left my skin sticky due to the humidity. My Mother joked that air conditioning made a relationship last and attraction followed.

My Mom pushed me to consume more calories, but food didn't interest me. Breaking one hundred pounds before the start of eleventh grade sounded impossible. Oh the hardship of being a skinny girl.

My Mom ate beside me, so I continued to eat. I realized she gained weight, while I remained as thin as ever. Maybe my fast metabolism kept me underweight. Due to my conditions, I required more energy to complete the same tasks.

The August after my surgery I saw Dr. Eduardo, who noticed I stayed rather lean. A growing girl should weigh more than ninety pounds. Dr. Eduardo suggested I dig into a poutine on the way home.

I asked what could be done to repair my ribs that stuck out in odd places. The doctor paused for a brief moment to collect his thoughts and apologized to me.

A silent water droplet slid down my cheek; followed by a few more in quick succession, but no sound came out of my mouth. A lone tear rolled down his overly tanned cheek and Dr. Eduardo whimpered as he excused himself to regain his composure.

I began to blubber into my Dad's chest. He rubbed my back, trying to ease my emotional pain. I didn't mean to make the doctor cry. He couldn't fulfill my request, so he felt badly.

In August, Olivia slept over. We fell asleep on the family room floor. We stomped upstairs for breakfast at ten thirty. We slumped onto the couch and woke up enough to get some food. Liv stood up and turned back to pull me up. My parents saw I'd be alright. My Dad set out two extra bowls of his famous fruit and oatmeal and the sweet aroma of warm berries wafted from the kitchen.

The summer weather gradually disappeared. My mother handed me a back to school flyer. I tucked my hair behind my ear and rolled my eyes in mock defiance.

*****

September arrived and I waited for my chemistry class to begin. The girl sitting in the seat behind me tapped my shoulder and I turned stiffly. She wondered what happened to my neck and I began to panic until I clued in. My surgical scar was showing above my collar. Relief flooded her face as she understood why the top of my spine glowed pink.

When school finished for the day, I threw my hood up and headed to the waiting minivan. Dr. Nasty expected me later on that afternoon. He never failed to brighten my day.

Dr. Nasty applied the usual neurological tests. I stood and closed my eyes. He moved behind me in case I completely lost my footing. Friedreich's Ataxia patients often lose their balance. The new residents watched what happened when I closed my eyes. As I lost my reference points I swayed back and forth, a telltale sign of Friedreich's Ataxia. Some of the residents freaked out a bit because most people control balance, even in the dark.

I turned sixteen in November, so Dr. Nasty gave me his email address. He expected me to continue to update him on my progress in between our appointments. I could email Dr. Nasty as questions arose about neurological stuff or life in general.

Dr. Nasty's faith in me, pushed me forward. I appreciated the invisible security blanket he provided. I moved onward and upward. Sometimes just knowing he believed in me got me through difficult times.

Throughout my first week back at school, I dropped my books on the floor by my locker frequently. Liv bent down and retrieved my binders and textbooks. At the start of the second week my notebook fell and I stared at the floor, willing the paperback into my hands. My muscles got stronger every day. I learned to pickup my books off the floor. I retrained my body. I appeared like a frog, but captured my agenda in my left hand and stood up. I ditched the old man grunt and smiled. I grabbed the horrible disorder by the collar and decided to fight.

I met Dr. Nasty for a checkup in December. The hospital volunteers decorated each clinic with Christmas trees and winter scenes painted on the windows. My parents and I sat down in the waiting area. In the hallway, we heard bells ring and a deep voice. I figured Santa Claus visited the in-patients.

Santa and his elves walked into the clinic where I sat. Santa belly laughed. His helper elf handed out candy canes and presents to all the boys and girls. I watched a magical scene unfold.

The elf brought over a gift. When I saw a walkman (the iPod of my day), a tear rolled down my cheek. The generosity touched my heart. I wanted a child to use the cassette player because I owned a similar one. Santa should see the little kids; I felt badly for taking a gift. The elf saw my Dad place the box back on top of Santa's sack of toys.

I looked around at all of the parents peering down at their happy wee tykes. An elf came over to us and handed me a large stuffed dog with a bone in his mouth and a big bag of toiletries for teens. We politely declined, but the elf insisted I keep the gifts. I cried silent tears. I thanked him multiple times.

I couldn't begin to tell you what happened at my clinic visit with Dr. Nasty. Perhaps he or Dr. Eduardo had something to do with Santa's visit. My parents and I were moved by the joy that filled the waiting room on that late December afternoon.

The opened boxes and happy faces spread across the room. I wished to handout toys around the holidays and make my heart sing. Receiving presents provided delight in the children's hearts including the teenagers.

Puzzle Pieces

The woman droned on. We parked for free on convocation day. The university rarely misses an opportunity to collect funds.

*****

Just before my eighteenth birthday in November, 2000, I asked Dr. Nasty what could be done to repair my protruding ribs. He referred me to an orthopedic surgeon. Hallelujah.

I started seeing an adult neurologist. I departed the safe environment of Dr. Nasty's clinic and entered a new medical office at the same hospital. I ought to have a doctor for adults, should I be in the hospital. Dr. Nasty matched me with the right doctor.

My parents and I stepped into a modern waiting room at the hospital, killing time before my first appointment with Dr. Alex Sutton. My Dad researched my new neuromuscular doctor and read some amazing accolades. Dr. Sutton sounded fabulous already and none of us laid eyes on him yet.

A young woman in her mid-twenties called my name and led through automatic double doors to an exam room. Gabrielle Iverson, the nurse practitioner for Dr. Sutton's clinic obtained my brief medical history.

On the way to the patient rooms I spotted offices, testing equipment, a giant accessible washroom, and lots of exam areas. Studies happened behind closed doors.

While we talked with Dr. Sutton, he stretched his arms and legs. His excess energy filled the spotless room.

Dr. Sutton told us Friedreich's Ataxia had no cure. Many treatments will work in combination to alleviate some symptoms of the disease. Some of the puzzle pieces are missing, but doctors worked on finding a solution.

He spoke the truth, but in an excited manner. The topic of a neuro-degenerative disorder could easily depressing, so I appreciated his tactfulness.

Once we finished chatting to Dr. Sutton, we talked to one of his medical coordinators. Daphne Tag co-ordinated some of the medical studies of the clinic. I felt connected to her right off the bat.

She handed me her business card in case I wanted to email any questions of my own. Somehow I knew Daphne and I would develop a friendship.

Daphne supplied a lot of information. She ran drug studies for certain disorders. She asked if I would partake in a research project where I became the subject. I supposed being involved in a study assisted the doctors in developing a cure. Daphne had no experiments pertaining to people with Friedreich's Ataxia, but one could materialize soon.

*****

During February of 2001, a phone message from Dr. David Torrent's office requested an appointment. I visited the adult orthopedic surgeon two weeks later. My life occurred at warp speed. I wished the doctor would agree to operate. I kept my fingers crossed. I anxiously awaited the doctor's entrance.

Dr. Torrent viewed my most recent x-rays. He could remove twenty percent of six ribs, so my back would lay flatter. He said the surgery may ease some of my shoulder pain, but he made no guarantees.

Dr. Torrent was dressed in preppy attire, a freshly pressed plaid shirt and flat front khaki pants. He could have been an 'Abercrombie & Fitch' model. My face lit up like a Christmas tree.

I wanted a straight back and a medical procedure seemed to be the best option. My Mom grinned at me. Hooray for surgery.

July couldn't come fast enough. My pre-op appointment eventually rolled around. My Mom and I met a nurse in a small room painted light green. "What are you having done Sweetie?" The middle-aged lady looked at me. Really? Did she not know the answer to her own question? "Thoroplasty of the right lumbar." Even after I explained the perplexed look on her face continued. I guessed the nurse had to assess my mental capabilities.

My surgery day came with the slowness of molasses. Blood work frightened me, but surgery transpired and I didn't panic. Macaroni and cheese and alphabet soup served up at the children's hospital, but not in the adult wing. Dry toast and beef broth made my post-op menu.

My surgery wrapped up and the doctor appeared to be pleased with the results. I touched my chapped lips. My mouth craved liquid and my back hurt. My eyes sealed shut with sleep. For someone who applied lip balm multiple times a day; dry cracked lips felt odd. What had I done?

My cousin Mary Pellic couldn't come to the hospital because her radiation zapped her energy. My Aunt Kayla came with gifts in tow. Mary made a card especially for me referring to a family joke. At a dinner a few months previous, the kids talked about celebrity crushes. I picked Jim Belushi because he was cute and real. Jim made me laugh on television. I found his chubby body attractive.

The card read: *Jim Belushi couldn't come and see you because he is taping a new sitcom. Jim sends his best.*

I laughed until I winced from pain. I couldn't believe I chose Jim Belushi over guys with a six pack of abs. I should have selected Leonardo DiCaprio or Brad Pitt.

My cousin, Norah Fairmont, came to visit me in the hospital. She stepped into my room and wrinkled her button nose at the horrid odor she breathed in. My dinner tray parked on my bedside table and the stench killed my appetite. Norah peered under the lid, allowing steam to rise and the disgusting aroma to permeate the sterile room. My meal resembled cat food. I dry heaved for a quick second, and then gulped the stale air, pushing away the food with my skinny little arms.

I wished I qualified for a kid's menu. Macaroni and cheese stayed in my brain, but alas I just turned nineteen. I longed for the warm cheesy goodness, like a warm hug from my Mom.

After a summer of recovery my parents and I travelled to the hospital for a post-op check-up. The waiting room smelled like freshly buttered toast.

Dr. Torrent peeked at my back. The results far exceeded his expectations and some swelling remained. My Mom thought Dr. Torrent should call his mother to inform her, medical school had been worth every penny. He was a fabulous surgeon.

*****

October brought cooler weather. I tried to be optimistic. My life could have been a lot worse. I a glanced around the lobby of the children's hospital and realized I was one of the fortunate ones. My Mom says I was her healthiest child. How sad. She referred to the fact I caught a cold infrequently. I'd be a shoe in for the child with the weirdest ailments. Dark humour got me through tough situations.

By this point, I experienced depressed moods a fair bit. Chad and Nicole suggested conferring with a psychologist might assist me in altering my frame of mind. Nicole told me therapy would teach me how to deal with what depresses me. A lot of people go to a psychologist or counselor in order to improve their outlook on life.

I decided seeing a shrink would be a great idea. I needed step by step instructions on what to do next. Chad recommended I email Dr. Nasty. His advice improved my disposition.

Dear Dr. Nasty,
I'm not sure how to handle all of the emotions building up beneath my calm exterior.
After my diagnosis with the help of some physiotherapy, my body seemed to rebound and walking became easier. As my body started to decline; my spirits have plummeted.
My body is betraying me, slowly, but surely. What do I do from here on out?
Thank you so much for all you do.
Megan McIntyre

In the meantime, my brother and sister-in-law said I could discuss any issues with our family friend Denise Pinot. Her background in psychology made delving into my problems a lot easier. Other people felt down in the dumps on occasion too and my health exacerbated my emotions. Denise thought I'd benefit from visiting a psychologist.

I heard the ping alerted me to a new email; I carefully transferred myself from my bed to my desk chair. I blinked at my laptop, rubbing sleep from my eyes, so I focused on the screen.

Dear Megan,
Coming to terms with a diagnosis is never as straight forward as we'd like it to be. I'm glad you felt comfortable enough to ask for help. I know that is hard for you to do.
Try to remember that a diagnosis isn't a prognosis.
I propose sitting down with a psychologist. You've studied psychology, so you know the advantages of therapy.
With your approval, I'll speak to Dr. Sutton and we'll match you with a psychologist. I have someone in mind I think you'll like.
Let me know what you prefer and we'll get the ball rolling.
Cheers,

Rowan R. Nasty

I supposed he wasn't wrong. My parents read the email and expressed their support in whatever option I decided on.

Dear Dr. Nasty,
Thank you so much for lending a hand. I'd like to see a psychologist. I think
that given my circumstances, it would be good for me to unload so to speak.
I'd be glad of your assistance in finding the right psychologist for me.
Thank you so much.
Megan McIntyre

Time seemed to be going by in slow motion. The next week I received mail from the hospital.

October, 2001
Dear Megan McIntyre,
This letter is to inform you of your appointment with Dr. Philip Gowan, a
psychologist who works out of McMaster University Medical Center.
Your appointment is the first Tuesday of November at 12 noon.
His office is located in the yellow section of the main floor, department 2Q.

Dr. Gowan introduced himself and wheeled me back to an office. I used a wheelchair full-time now, as my legs could no longer support my body.

During my first appointment I would get to know Dr. Gowan and figure out if our styles meshed. I pictured a dark cherry sofa made of tufted leather with rounded edges in a walnut paneled office. I thought the patient lay down and spilled their guts. I sat on a bright purple couch across from the doctor. Pictures of fruit decorated the office walls.

He informed me the first couple of visits usually dug up some raw emotions. Once we got to know each other a bit better, our appointments would be less stressful. Dr. Gowan worked with both teenagers and adults, so we got along just fine.

Dr. Nasty selected by Dr. Gowan especially for me. I didn't know either of my grandpas, but Dr. Gowan seemed the epitome of what I imagined a grandfather to be. His beard reminded me of Santa Claus. He calmed my frayed nerves.

*****

Dr. Sutton had some news about a drug study for people with Friedreich's Ataxia. I previously agreed to participate in any research pertaining to my disorder. Now the question became whether I would fit within the parameters set by the drug companies.

My parents and I sat in a small office with a desk and four office chairs. I hoped Daphne didn't invite more patients. The whole process of a drug study was new to us.

Daphne did a bunch of neurological tests and near the end Gabrielle came in to draw my blood. Dr. Sutton consulted with Daphne in the hallway before he entered the room. He repeated a few simple activities to assess my fine motor skills.

I met the criteria for the medical testing. The research involved weekly blood samples and taking orange goo twice a day. The cough syrup like substance didn't have a pleasant taste. The research was a double-blind study. Meaning some of the clients received a placebo, some assigned a lighter version of the drug, and others got a high dose. The participants never knew what dosage they got.

I saw Dr. Gowan every Tuesday at noon.

My Dad told me if I didn't know someone, one way to get to know a person, was to ask them a question. Dr. Gowan asked all of the questions. A one sided conversation became second nature after a while.

Dear Daphne,
I really don't like liquid medicine, but I have managed to get most of the orange junk in my mouth and swallow.
See you on Tuesday at the crack of 11:30AM.
Megan

*****

December came in with a lot of snow and blustery days. I came to McMaster to see my shrink. My parents consumed hot chocolate in the hospital café.

I wanted to blend into the background of my life and being a disabled made invisibility somewhat impossible. When I required assistance, I felt like my disability won a battle. I wasn't going to let my deteriorating abilities take over my life.

Dr. Gowan made my muddled mind clear. Being invisible had downfalls too. How would anybody notice an imperceptible human? I concentrated on what I could do. He said, asking for assistance shouldn't be seen as a sign of defeat. My wheelchair was a tool to let me conquer the world, or at least the accessible parts.

So what if I'd never go up or down a set of stairs ever again. Between elevators and lifts I wouldn't be missing out on much. Stairs could be a pain in the ass most of the time anyway. I think anybody who has ever gone barefoot down a set of stairs and stepped on a piece of Lego would agree with me.

A new year had begun and therapy sessions carried on. I attempted to dump a week's worth of troubles in sixty minutes. Dr. Gowan initiated a topic and I tried to figure out what the subliminal message meant. When he asked what television shows I watched, I was confused.

I watched medical dramas and crime shows. Reality television made me see my own life in a positive light. I found reality shows to be similar to a soap opera. For an hour I could immerse myself into the characters. While watching television shows I didn't think about my own issues. In some cases after watching a show I believed my life passed for normal.

My favourite way to spend time didn't include reflecting on my own life. I wasn't comfortable with my inner self. When I stopped to contemplate my own life, I often got tears in the corner of my eyes.

Young adults didn't consider wheelchairs, medication, doctors and physiotherapy usual topics. A conversation with older teenagers usually involved talk of dating, education, and careers.

I continued the weekly blood draws before I met with Dr. Gowan for the research project. I prayed the results would lead to a breakthrough. Surely somebody could find a way to put the disgusting liquid into a gel cap.

By the time February rolled into town, Dr. Gowan had me thinking beyond my appointment time. He knew how to get to the heart of the matter without prying into my existence. I was fascinated by observing him in his natural habitat.

Dr. Gowan wondered if I wanted to see him less often. The thought terrified me. The rhythm of our time together established a nice routine. He nodded and never discussed it again.

I didn't know what dosage I'd been assigned for the drug study. I tried not to think too much.

I noticed a sharp decline in my hand-eye coordination. Simple tasks like typing an email or picking up a pill became more difficult. Being kicked out of the program wasn't a situation I'd deal well with, so I remained mute on the subject.

While at my best friend Olivia's house, her father observed my decreasing coordination. Up until that moment, I imagined only a good outcome. I pushed the obvious changes out of my mind.

The next day, my parents and I put our heads together. My parents spotted negative changes as well. We had to speak to Daphne at the next study appointment.

The project approached the midway point and all the clients completed some extra testing. I picked up a round peg and put it in a circular hole. The peg board appeared large, but in reality the board spanned five by five. Twenty five pegs seemed excessive, but I drudged onward. The little sticks slipped out of my hands many times.

Daphne watched me complete the peg exercise and I could see the worry in her eyes. The sticks resembled a suppository. For all the good those pegs did, I may as well have shoved them up my ass.

Daphne informed my parents and I other people on the mystery drug experienced a loss of some coordination. Relief spread across my body and I confessed to running into problems. Daphne likely observed my somewhat rapid decline.

I believe I received the full strength dose. Due to the developing issues, those on the high portion would no longer be able to be subjects in the research. I jumped for joy because I swallowed the last of the icky medicine.

A high concentration of the medicine acted similar to having too many cups of coffee. Some people find one or two cups of coffee boosts energy. Drinking seven cups of coffee provided too many stimulants. The mystery drug acted in much the same way. More research should be completed, on how the smallest amount of the gloppy medicine reacted in Friedreich's Ataxia patients.

I weighed seventy two pounds at the start of the ninth grade. I differed both physically and mentally.

The doctor's eyes bugged out in concern, as thoughts of the eating disorders clinic he worked for overtook his mind. I was always told that I had a fast metabolism. I was never diagnosed with an eating disorder. I would be honest if I had. Many kids had made up their minds that I was anorexic. Depriving me of food wasn't even on my radar. My Mom always tried to put weight on me with ice cream, smoothies, and cheesy fries, but I remained a skinny kid.

I'd always just eaten what I wanted, when I wanted. And no matter what I ate, I didn't seem to gain much weight. At the time, I weighed around 110 pounds and was a little less than 5'7. Dr. Gowan wanted me to put on some weight. I lost myself in a sea of ice-cream, donuts, and smoothies.

*****

My neighbour's daughter, Addison Layton, took her master's at McMaster University and she sometimes came home with us after my visits with Dr. Gowan.

Dear Megan,
Are you at McMaster next Tuesday afternoon? I have a break between my classes and thought we could catch up since I'm not going home with you this week.
If you are, would you want to meet for hot chocolate in the café? Minnie makes the best hot chocolate around.
Thanks.
Your Neighbour,
Addison Layton

Dr. Gowan listened to my rambling conversations and allowed me to refresh my brain each week. My mental health rose up on days I spoke to my shrink. Talking to someone besides my parents expanded my comfort level with other persons. After my session with Dr. Gowan, my parents and I scouted out an empty table near where Addie usually came from.

Addie and I chatted like long lost best friends. I talked for an hour straight to Dr. Gowan, so at times I spoke very little. Addie chattered and filled in the silent gaps.

Addie knew I had weekly appointments at McMaster Children's Hospital, but she likely assumed the doctor visits pertained to the drug research I participated in. Most Tuesdays I saw the nurse for lab work, followed by a therapy session. However, I failed to disclose the fact I saw a psychologist. Addie procured the lead on our discussions; my mouth dry from chitchat to Dr. Gowan.

The drug study finished and yet I missed my friendship with Daphne. Our personalities clicked from our first conference. Fate brought us together for a reason and now the connection floated away.

Dear Megan,
Next Tuesday, after your appointment with Dr. Gowan are you & your parents available to meet for hot chocolate in the lobby café?
Our friendship shouldn't dissolve because you aren't in the study anymore. I hope I don't come off as weird.
Daphne

*****

By March, Dr. Gowan's happiness swelled once I gained a couple pounds. I became disheartened I couldn't eat whatever I chose, whenever I craved a snack. My inner self danced when I realized I fulfilled my final food diary.

Dear Daphne,
We must be have the same type of odd personalities because I had also been hoping our friendship didn't have to come to an abrupt halt once the project closed. Hot chocolate would be nice. See you on Tuesday about 1 o'clock.
Megan

*****

Dr. Gowan addressed my parents and me at the end of one of my appointments regarding his own health. He read the worried expression on my face. His oncologist diagnosed his headaches as a rare cancer. Surgery on his brain left a shaved area on the back of his head. Dr. Gowan cancelled a small number of scheduled dates because of his radiation time table, but he committed to his patients.

I tried to keep my sniffles to a minimum, but that was next to impossible.

We met with Daphne for a warm drink. The hot chocolate and conversation brought sunshine to our hearts on an otherwise gloomy day.

Megan,
I'm sorry that we weren't able to meet this week. I hope you don't mind that I got your email address from Dr. Nasty.
I trust your week is going well. I'll have access to my email, so feel free to drop me a line.
Dr. P. Gowan

April Fools brought me a cold, but I laughed little. I stayed home on Tuesday to be considerate of Dr. Gowan's already compromised state.

Dr. Gowan phoned because he heard I caught a bug. He checked on my mental clarity. Plugged sinuses meant my facial muscles hurt, but I managed to keep in positive mood. My sore throat made my voice sound groggy.

One morning in May, I rolled over and rubbed my sleepy eyes. My parents leaned on either side of my bedroom door frame. By the concern showing in their eyes, I figured something must be amiss. I sat up clutching my flannel covered knees and gently rocked myself back and forth.

*****

Dr. Nasty called and left a message for me to phone him back. I wondered why the urgency to speak to me. My calendar displayed nothing about seeing Dr. Nasty. I supposed the call could prove to be about Dr. Gowan. I was scheduled to meet my shrink at noon.

Dr. Gowan died during the night. His illness made him slow down, but only for a week or two. Grief overtook my mind. I presumed his health would improve.

I froze in place. A lone tear fell down my face followed by many more. My mother stroked my hair as the morning sunshine came in between the slats of my blinds covering my window.

I barely spoke, raw feelings filled my heart. I figured Dr. Nasty kept to his schedule and eventually we'd connect. When I identified myself and the secretary put me through to Dr. Nasty himself, I felt special. I already knew Dr. Nasty to be an amazing doctor, but the call proved he had a heart of gold.

Whenever Dr. Nasty ran into Dr. Gowan, he always mentioned me. Nasty connected us and I will be forever grateful for the introduction to therapy. Dr. Gowan and Dr. Nasty met at work and became fast friends.

Dr. Nasty wanted to catch me before we left to come to the hospital. I sniffled and attempted desperately not to break into a sobbing mess. His voice wrapped around me like a hug.

Dr. Nasty comforted me and I him. I offered to go to the funeral visitation. Dr. Nasty thought the Gowan family would appreciate me doing so. Dr. Nasty promised to let me know the funeral arrangements as soon as the family had finalized the plans.

Dr. Gowan had a heart attack at his office late the previous night. By the time the emergency people got to him, too much time had passed since his last breath.

Dr. Nasty said once everything settled down, he and I could speak about continued therapy. I pressed the end button on the portable phone and remained in the quiet of the spring morning.

My shrink died. My life sounded like a Hallmark made for television movie. Maybe I should write a book…

I turned to my mother and silently cried into her shoulder.

Dr. Nasty went above and beyond what anyone expected. When you look up the word gem in the dictionary, Dr. Nasty's photo should be beside the definition.

I couldn't start fresh and explain my life to someone new. Dr. Gowan and I had an easy relationship. Dr. Gowan's advice lived on in my head, stored away for me to reflect on the lessons he taught me.

The children's hospital I went to hosted a telethon each spring to raise funds for new equipment and renovations. Dr. Gowan had been interviewed about the new youth development clinic being opened in the summer. I found the clip on the internet and watched Dr. Gowan speak multiple times. Each time I heard his soothing voice I wished to pull him out of my computer monitor and hug him until he was well again.

I trusted Dr. Gowan looked down on his family and friends. I felt better knowing that illness couldn't survive in Heaven.

I strongly disliked change.

Time marched on. I decided whether to sit down on the sideline and watch life pass me by, or find my place and join in. I appreciated my existence because of therapy.

Thank you Dr. Gowan.

Family

I appeared dazed as I zoned in and out of my graduation ceremony. I drifted from the present day to far back into my childhood. I remembered a lot, so when I dreamed about the past, the scene occurred the same way.

*****

My Mom was my best friend. We spent a lot of time together each day whether we read or watched television, we always managed to squeeze every last moment of fun out of our down periods. Occasionally we hit a bumpy patch, but we worked our differences out.

My Mom and I like a lot of the same activities, so we get along well. We both enjoy scrapbooking our photos. My Mom and I found pleasure in our family and friends.

My Dad and I have a complex relationship. Our personalities could be similar, so we try to win the argument. Once we let things permeate, one of us backs down and we go happily along.

My Dad sat in my corner, regardless of any squabbles on a given day. I continued to be his little princess, baby and pumpkin, all rolled into one. My household never had a shortage of affection.

As far back as I can recall my parents showed affection to each other, to my two older brothers and me. Every night we tell each other we love one another. Ending the day on a positive note made falling asleep easier.

I learned to read for leisure. My parents read the paper and each had a novel on the go. Our family subscribed to several magazines. My Mother and Father led by example. Books allowed an escape to the other side of the world or any setting you imagined.

My father read me books from his childhood. I touched the yellow stained paper because the faded pages were a connection to my Dad's younger years. I resembled a wee princess snuggled against his side while I listened to his deep voice.

My Dad wore glasses when he read. I wondered what he viewed. I plopped down next to my Dad and tried to catch a glimpse of what he saw. I annoyed him a small bit, but we usually ended our chats with laughter.

*****

Family had constantly been important to my parents. My father was one of fifteen first cousins on his paternal lineage. Almost every summer we went to a reunion of the McIntyre and Heartline family descendants. A number of my father's first cousins became farmers in the village of Campden. My Dad's generation invited their kids and grandchildren. On the day of the get-together, every available family member headed out to one of the farms for a Sunday afternoon picnic.

My mother happily refers to the outing as the McHeartline Picnic. A pig roasted on a spit because some of the farmers raised hogs. My Dad's oldest cousin, Trevor Heartline, prepares corn on his steam engine. Everybody brings a salad or dessert and lawn chairs. We ate and conversed into the evening.

I hardly ever missed the family picnic. I had plenty of playmates. Mitchell and Violet's daughter Ivy and I often amused ourselves. Our parents snapped photos of the two of us standing in a wash tub filled with water at about age three. We both wore ruffled bathing suits because people wore swim outfits in a pool. Ivy and I engaged in recreational activities with the other cousins.

The grandchildren played together in a giant sandbox or swimming pool, depending on which farm the gathering took place. The city kids got a look at farm life. Squeals of laughter and the odd cry after a scraped knee, but by and large the kids remained content in the absence of electronic tablets or toys.

One year a blow up bouncy castle for the kids to run and jump all afternoon. Needless to say, the children kept busy and entertained for most of the day. Parents and grandparents beamed happiness because their offspring went home exhausted. My Dad's cousin Mitchell and his wife Violet bounced around before too many kids took over the air filled palace.

Since the reunions generally happened a year apart, I watched the children grow up right before my eyes. Now we wore name tags, so everyone could recognize the names. A few new babies arrived each year.

*****

My Mom was an only child. She had two cousins on her mother's side which we saw sporadically. On her father's line lots of cousins existed, but we saw them infrequently. No major event that caused us to stop seeing each other; we became spread out and lead hectic lives with our respective families.

On my father's maternal side he had nineteen first cousins including his siblings and himself. I grew up going to Sterling family bridal showers. The aunts of my grandmother's generation put on a shower for the kids of my father's era.

The custom passed on to the next generation, hosted by the aunts of my mother's age group. A number of years nobody got married, so I longed for tea, cake and the companionship of the strong ladies in my family. A few skipped the Sterling family shower. The tradition began to slide away.

We have recently had a family bridal shower, so I am hoping the practice is revived. As a small girl I remember being with all of the women in my extended family and being in awe the happenings around me. I prayed one day the bridal shower would be thrown in my honour.

*****

My Dad was close to his siblings. My Auntie Leona and Uncle Ted Fairmont turned out to be the closest geographically, so we tended to see more of them throughout the years. Norah Fairmont and I happened to be the youngest two of our McIntyre cousins, so we shared a lot of memories.

I was one of ten McIntyre grandchildren. I spent more time with some of my cousins, depending on the amount of contact. I used emails, texting social media to stay up to date on family goings on. Norah and I carried on being, best friends.

Before I came on the scene, the McIntyre extended family started gathering on the weekend before Christmas for dinner and mingling. The hosting task rotated between the four McIntyre children.

We used to hold the family Christmas potluck at each of the family homes, but now we often had the event at a hotel. All of the food prep and cleanup by the venue staff, so we could focus on socializing with relatives. Our family kept growing and nobody had space to seat upwards of thirty people for dinner.

Norah brought her boyfriend Lucas to family Christmas. Luke seemed nice enough. I'd met Luke at a dinner at my Auntie Leona and Uncle Ted's home and he presented himself well.

My cousin Ellie was roughly ten years older than me. Our fathers were brothers. My Uncle Noah passed away in 1997, after a courageous battle with colon cancer. My Aunt Lily became widow. She continued to be a part of our family. Once I was an adult, she said I didn't need put aunt in front of her name. When I email my Aunt I call her A. L., but I refused to drop the word aunt completely.

Ellie entertained Norah and me when we attended family functions years ago. Now we connect through email and chat about writing and life in general.

Ellie had two teenage daughters who occupied the younger kids. Stephanie and Maeve Tucker showed up ready to work with the younger cousins at the arts and craft table.

One of Ellie's teenaged daughters, Maeve Tucker, played travel hockey for a Stoney Creek team. Her other daughter Stephanie preferred to write, so we linked up on social media or at the hockey arena.

My parents and I had just got home from my Aunt Nina and Uncle Russell's family Christmas party in Bancroft. Norah phoned at about 11 o'clock. Immediately I worried an accident had transpired. She sounded breathless, but somehow she managed to squeeze out that Lucas proposed.

*****

My parents tried to meet Norah's family at our Grandma McIntyre' house. Norah and I fooled around together while the adults caught up. We explored the bedroom cupboards full of toys accumulated through the years. When we got older we went to the park around the corner by ourselves.

I didn't mind sitting with the grown-ups. My Grandma had a painting hung over her couch. The art landscape of a northern forest in the fall provided me hours of imaginative fun. When I was the only child, I went on a hike through the forest and visualized the trees around myself.

When the time came to divide up my Grandma McIntyre' belongings, the painting stood leaning against my parents' dining room wall, because nobody had a spot for the picture. When I recalled my memories of the artwork, my parents' decided to keep the painting. I cherished my fond remembrances. I expected the colourful artwork to be passed on within my family, alongside the story.

*****

When I was about 8 years old, I had a sleepover at my Grandma McIntyre' home my Grandpa built. My Grandma kept talking about her sister Billie's male friend being a saint. I had met Aunt Billie, but couldn't recall a man with an aura of an angel surrounding him.

When I returned home, I questioned my parents about the new word I learned. They defined the word saint as a person who does good deeds throughout their life. In my Grandma's mind, Nicholas was a saint for putting on a smile and keeping Billie out of trouble.

I wondered why my Great Aunt Billie had a name more typical of a boy. Her real name was Wilhelmina, but her whole family thought she was going to be a boy. Everyone referred to her as Billie, instead of her real name.

My parents made family a priority and expectations trickled down to my brothers and me. My Dad and Uncle Noah started our family tree after I toddled into their lives. When my Uncle Noah passed away, my Dad kept researching and adding to our ancestral roots. My Dad found the process interesting and one day my brothers and I would join in the pursuit.

Toys

My bum started to go numb. I had the added gel cushion of my wheelchair. The rest of the auditorium sat in a stacking chair made of unforgiving wood, so I didn't fidget or protest to my neighbours.

I resumed my search for my childhood recollections.

*****

I was blessed with a family who sees me as a person and not a disability. As a child I loved crafting and imaginative play. Being the only girl in my family, I by no means lacked attention. Since my brothers came a long while before me, I call myself a bonus child.

I flashed back to Christmastime when I just turned two years old. I became the center of my family's universe. Even though I didn't say much, my family still watched my every move.

Audrey Porter, maternal grandmother, got so much merriment out of shopping for me. I was her only granddaughter. I was the ninth grandchild of Naomi McIntyre. During wakeful instances, I only stopped for quick snuggle periodically, before I insisted on running. My grandmothers took pleasure when I let them smell the baby lotion on my skin.

*****

Winter got colder and colder, the boys joked around inside. A few kids had come over to hang out with my brothers in the family room. I went down the stairs slowly. Our neighbour Tessa Carpini often engaged me in an activity. Chad handed me a note I took upstairs to our mother.

Dear Mom,
Can you keep her upstairs please?
She's BUGGING us.

Will, Chad & Guests

I couldn't read. I irritated the boys. My Mom distracted me with books. My Mom brought me a cookie in the shape of a maple leaf.

*****

Our Christmas tree down and all of the decorations put in the basement. January of 1985 was an exciting time for my family. I got to meet my new baby cousin. My Auntie Leona and Uncle Ted adopted a baby girl. I considered myself a big girl, or so I thought. My Mom and I went to the toy store to adopt a baby doll.

I was curious if Auntie Leona and Uncle Ted went to the toy store too. I grew in my Mommy's tummy, but I didn't comprehend the word adoption. My Mom explained my baby cousin grew inside another lady's tummy. Auntie Leona and Uncle Ted dreamed of a baby girl so much that another lady shared her baby with them.

The words didn't quite fit together in my head. I had to inquire about getting a 'liddle sister'. I was the last baby my parents would have.

The toy store contained aisles of dolls all waiting to be adopted. My senses overwhelmed by the choices and I gazed from side to side. My Mom coached me toward the right section of the store.

I pointed to the red haired Cabbage Patch Kid wearing a pair of yellow corduroy overalls, with a white ruffle trimmed blouse underneath. My mother picked up the box as I hopped up and down in agreement.

On January 24th 1985, my family and I went to meet the new baby. I carried my new doll with pride. My Uncle Ted had shoveled the snow to the side of the driveway. We walked up to my Auntie Leona and Uncle Ted front door. The sun streamed through the glass outer door.

I wondered where my aunt and uncle hid the baby. My Dad slipped off my boots and put on pink ballet slippers I had received for my birthday. Auntie Leona put her finger to her lips and we followed her down the hall to the baby's room.

Will picked me up and set me on his hip, so I could see the sleeping baby in her crib. "That's a pretty baby," I mumbled to myself. Her name was Norah Brooklyn Fairmont. Auntie Leona stared at her two week old baby girl with happiness oozing from her body.

Chad shared his birthday with Norah's adoption day. We had a lot to

51

celebrate. We headed to the living room to let Norah sleep a while longer.

Auntie Leona directed us to the dusty rose sofas. The new furniture looked great in their living room. When they knew Norah was coming, my Auntie Leona asked my Mom if she'd go with her to buy some clothing for the baby. They ended up getting the couches in addition to some sleepers.

Leona touched my doll on the arm, wondering her name. I introduced Miriam, perking up from my seat. I told Auntie Leona I adopted her from the store. A lone tear ran down my Auntie Leona's right cheek. She thought Norah and I would be best friends.

My Auntie Leona was right; Norah and I became the best of friends. Norah was meant to be a part of our family. Fate brought us together, but family kept us together.

*****

I tired of winter easily. Snowsuits involved a lot of work to go outside. Finally the sun came out to play in April.

Spring arrived after an extended winter. My mother stepped up into the living room with an armful of clean, unfolded towels to see me peering out the bay window on my tiptoes. I saw sunshine and my boys.

I could hardly wait to play outside when my brothers got home from school. My mother folded another kitchen towel. I intended to ride my bike. I stamped my feet with enthusiasm.

Miriam the Cabbage Patch Doll seemed to hold a permanent spot on my hip. I noticed how parents and other adults picked up their babies.

My mother stood to go put the dish towels away. The boys came in and noticed a plate of maple leaf cookies on the kitchen table. The boys offered to take me out front for some fresh air. My excess energy continued to develop into the early afternoon because the rain kept me indoors.

Chad popped a cookie in his mouth and grasped my little hand. Our neighbour Tessa Carpini was coming over to see me after she dropped her back pack off at home. Chad opened the garage door so I could get my tricycle out, and any other outdoor toys we wished to amuse ourselves with. My mother gave a grateful smile to the boys as she started to fold the large bath towels.

I had to listen to my brothers and Tessa. I had to try to keep Miriam out of the puddles. I tugged at Chad's arm and off we went. Tessa made her way across our crescent, skipping with each step. We waved at her until she caught sight of us.

My bike was stuck in the garage, so Will jumped in and retrieved it. I sat down on the white seat, placing Miriam between myself and the handlebars. Will didn't see that ending well for Miriam. Chad agreed, but I rarely did anything without a doll by my side.

Tessa stopped skipping at the end of our driveway to lend me a hand in turning around. I happily complied, as I repositioned my doll. Tessa clapped her hands for my benefit.

My brothers and Tessa watched my doll drop from her position on the tricycle to the blacktop in slow motion. I was too shocked to do anything but cry out.

Will rushed to my side and saw no scrapes on me. He had a look at Miriam's face. Will went inside to clean the doll up and get a band aid.

Will cleaned Miriam up as best he could, but the skid mark on her cheek remained. Will figured a band aid would make her boo boo all better. What a good big brother. My Mom had been sorting and putting away laundry while the boys tired me out. She had a look at the doll and lovingly patted Will's shoulder. Will stayed calm during a disaster or a perceived medical issue.

Miriam was a brave patient. Will slowly handed the doll back to me. Miriam had a permanent skid mark on her face. I kissed her boo-boo and went on playing with my doll, lost in my own world of make believe.

I shouldn't bike on the street, so Chad and Tessa took me around the crescent on the sidewalk. Chad waved his hand approximating a checkered flag, like they used in car racing. My cabin fever cured for the moment.

*****

I had turned three during November. Christmas music saturated the air waves. My brothers and I to headed to bed so Santa Claus could come. My brothers long ago determined the role of Santa was carried out by Mom and Dad, but nobody cared to spoil the excitement for me.

Bed? How could I be expected to sleep? Santa and his reindeer landed in a neighbouring city. I turned around at the top of the stairs and said goodnight to my parents and Grandma Porter. My father peered up the stairs at me in my red, plaid pyjamas, the wavy collar askew. He busily wrapped the gifts he bought for my mother at the dining room table. I hadn't discovered my parents picking out their own gifts. Where's the surprise in that?

If my alarm clock started with a seven, we could wake up, but not before then. Unless an emergency occurred, our parents didn't wish to be disturbed before seven. The three of us kids flew up the stairs.

The boys agreed to come and wake me up when morning arrived and we could open presents. Chad used his right hand to mess my hair and I squirmed with delight.

On Christmas morning, Chad and Will waited patiently for the clock to reach seven. Chad rubbed my back until I began to stir.

I scurried to the top of the stairs and surveyed the vast array of presents. Wow. I stepped carefully down the stairs one at a time.

When everybody had their stocking and a comfy seat, we could begin opening the tissue covered packages that spilled onto the carpet. My Dad collected the crumpled, tissue paper for recycling.

My favourite candy was Smarties. I ripped off the last bit of tissue paper from the gigantic cardboard tube filled with my favourite treat. Chad opened a frosted mint chocolate bar tore the wrapper, bit a piece. Chocolate before breakfast? Will popped the lid off the chip container and ate a few chips before replacing the cap. Pringles are a staple in the stockings at our house. My parents had prepared a brunch. Chips and chocolate tasted so good in the early Christmas morning.

Gold coins hid in the toes of our stockings. Although technically the chocolate coins came from Santa, the boys had an inkling Grandma purchased the sweet treat. Little Miss Giggles, Santa had chosen the perfect book for me. My Mom promised to read it to me that night before I went to bed.

We always had bacon, eggs, breakfast sausage, and toast for breakfast when we were finished opening our stockings. My mother stared at my brothers and me with a hint of a grin appearing on her face.

Will and Chad found a present for everyone. Wrapping paper flew everywhere as I clawed the box open. "Fweepy." Will used scissors to pry off the ties holding the doll to the cardboard. Looking at the doll was like staring at a real toddler. I named her "Fweepy". The official title of the doll was Sleepy Real Baby.

I thanked my brother in my garbled three year old version of the English language.

Grandma got Chad a Nerf basketball net for his bedroom door. He blew her a thank you kiss from across the sea of wrapping paper. Chad balled up tissue paper and made a three point shot into the garbage bag my Dad held open.

Mom and Dad got Will a Toronto Blue Jays baseball hat. He put on his new hat and modeled for our parents. He looked goofy with the brim straight across, but he would curve the peak later.

I passed my Dad a present. I winked and went back to playing with my new doll. He unwrapped the parcel ever so slowly because he figured I picked out the gift.

He pulled on the blond leather gloves and beamed from ear to ear.

"They ought to be nice because Mommy paid fifty dollars." I blurted out the price. Everyone began to laugh and I amused myself in the middle of my new toys.

My eyes glanced out the bay window, watched big fluffy flakes tumble down onto our blacktop driveway. The scene was like a Norman Rockwell painting. In fact, Santa brought us a puzzle of a poster he completed years ago. Usually a puzzle was under our Christmas tree for the whole family. We love traditions.

*****

In January of the following year our routines got back to day to day business. My Mom and I had a list of errands to run while the boys attended school. My Dad tiptoed out the door sometime after the sunrise, so he could work in quiet. If I behaved, we'd get a treat when we concluded.

I could only bring one doll out at a time, so I chose to bring Fweepy. I grabbed the doll by the hand and dragged her over to the stairs where my Mom bundled me up for the near freezing temperature outside.

First, we returned some library books and picked out some new bedtime stories. Hugga Bunch, the movie never disappointed me. My mother settled me on her hip to keep me out of the brown sugar-like slush that formed on the library parking lot. The library staff required indoor voices, so the study zone remained peaceful. Once we entered the lobby, I walked holding my mother's hand.

My Mom noticed patrons staring at her with horror in their eyes. Once my mother glanced in my direction, she realized why people judged her. 'Fweepy' felt heavy, so I dragged the doll across the terracotta tiles. As if my mother would let me lug a real baby by the arm socket.

My Mom wasn't a huge fan of Hugga Bunch, because I viewed it so many times. The content was a little weird, but the story was almost believable.

I pointed to the book on the display in the children's department of the library. Harry the Dirty Dog ranked among one of my favourite books.

Our errands finished, so my Mom and I headed over to the coffee shop for a donut. Later, we collected my brothers at school dismissal time. Sprinkle donuts reminded me of going to the coffee shop with my Mom. Running around town from store to store often ended in sharing a snack of some sort.

*****

My Aunt Leona and Uncle Ted babysat me one weekend. I posed a million questions and preferred to be active. My aunt was getting a snack ready while I went through Norah's toy box. When she asked me to choose how I would like to eat my banana, she expected my answer to be, sliced in a dish or divided in half.

I briefly paused my play. "I'd like my banana monkey style please." My Aunt understood exactly what I meant, even though she'd not heard my phrasing before.

*****

I grumbled while my Mom zipped up my puffy coat and slipped my feet into my warm boots. The boys arrived at the front door, backpacks in tow a moment later. The boys shouldn't walk to school in slush and ice, so Mom drove them. Grown-ups frowned upon kids staying home alone, so I tagged along.

*****

In March, my mother prepared for the coming Easter. When prompted, I told my Mom I liked Smarties. A soft and squishy stuffed animal made the top of my list.

While in the checkout line at the local Hallmark store, my mother spotted a whole display of stuffed toys. An employee offered to help. The lady pointed to a stuffed platypus that was soft and squishy. My Mom went in the card shop for stamps and checked another item off her list.

The Easter Bunny came. I sat up, wearing my fuzzy pink sleepers. Will fixed my hair before we went downstairs. I tried to see what my brother was doing, but gave up.

We had a happy Easter indeed. I shrieked at the sight of a solid white chocolate bunny leaning against my Easter basket. I pulled pink tissue paper out of a pastel purple gift bag with coloured Easter eggs on the front of it. I vibrated. A soft and squishy animal, just what I desired.

I didn't know a platypus until my Dad confirmed by reading the tag. The boys gave a slight smile toward their mother while I fooled around with my new stuffed animal friend. Chad spiked the fur of the platypus. I named her Platty. I peered at my new playmate with a fondness in my heart.

"Are going to see Grandma today?" I gazed up at my parents, sitting on our living room couch.

"Which Grandma are you referring to?" My Dad pitched the question to me.

"White Grandma." I answered somewhat irritated.

"What's your other Grandma called?" The humour in my Dad's face became evident.

"Black Grandma." I replied in frustration.

My brothers and parents attempted to suppress laughter. I distinguished my grandmothers based on their hair colour. Grandma Porter arrived in the early afternoon. Grandma McIntyre expected us and all of my cousins the next day.

I would get to be beside Norah. My sister. In reality Norah was my cousin. We slept over at our Grandma's house; we traveled together, and talked about stuff nobody else understood.

I even spent the night at Norah's other grandparents' house. I called them Grandma and Grandpa and no one corrected me, so I imagined us as sisters or sister-cousins.

On one occasion when Norah and I acted goofy upstairs in the 'girl's room' at our Grandma's house, she mentioned I didn't have a grandpa. She reached for the teddy bear, whose fur was the colour of peanut butter, and stated that I could share her Grandpa. My eyes overflowed in dramatic fashion.

My vision of a grandfather was a mix between Grandpa Fairmont and my best friend's grandpa, Hop. Both men remembered my Grandpa fondly. I craved a connection to my grandfather. Grandpa Fairmont and Hop made the image of my grandfather complete.

*****

Later that spring, we got a yellow lab puppy. She wasn't an ordinary pup though. My family was raising her to be a seeing eye dog for a blind person.

We all walked around in a happy daze. We named the dog Bixby. When my Dad brought her home, the dog and I were similar sizes. Her tail whipped around faster than I liked, but she was ecstatic to meet everyone.

Bixby had a lot to learn in a short amount of time. She wasn't perfect. One evening we came home to remnants of my doll family strewn about the living room. A yellow dress laid on the entrance hall carpet. The Heart Family couldn't be saved. I crossed my arms and stuck out my bottom lip.

Bixby didn't wait too long before she got herself into a bad situation. She bit the fingers of my beloved 'Sleepy Real Baby'. Fweepy performed the same. My brothers put pencils in the holes the dog left and labelled the doll "Freddie Kruger". I remember crying because the doll frightened me.

Bixby ate a few plants from our vegetable garden before she grew out of her puppy phase. As Bixby matured, she seemed to recognize she had an important job to do.

At the end of our year together, we had to send Bixby to the training center, where she would be matched to a blind person. Her paws left lasting impressions on all of our hearts.

If Bixby didn't do well in training center, we had the option of keeping her. My family wanted our girl to pass, but secretly we all hoped we'd get to be her forever home.

The invitation to Bixby's graduation stated the date, time and address. The card stock failed to note Bixby's status, but we assumed the commencement ceremony meant she moved forward to be a guide dog.

My family and I piled in our car on the day of Bixby's graduation and headed to the center. My Mom prepared my brothers and me for the moment our eyes locked on Bixby. When her harness was in place, we couldn't pet Bixby or distract her in any way.

"We're here to see Bixby." My mother found out directions from an information attendant. The rest of the family looked around at the many dogs alongside their new owners. When Bixby heard her name, she perked up, still in her harness.

We gathered around Bixby and her leader. My family and I cried silent tears. We met Isabelle, Bixby's new partner in crime. As introductions happened, Isabelle's eyes began to water and drip down her face. My brothers and I quietly blubbered in the corner. Isabelle was totally blind, but she sensed our raw emotions. My parents felt a connection to her.

Isabelle unhooked Bixby's working harness and the dog transformed into our contented puppy. Although six months lapsed between when we dropped Bixby off at training, she remembered all of us. I stood beside Bixby and put my little arms around her. In return she slobbered kisses all over my face, in the manner she often did at our house.

Chad excused himself and locked himself in our car. Bixby not only accomplished her intense training, received the valedictorian award. The Lions Foundation of Canada Dog Guides used her in the video given to people who expressed interest in raising a puppy for a year.

My family couldn't believe how attached we became to Bixby. We fulfilled our commitment to bring up a puppy for the seeing-eye dog program. Leaving the graduation reception without Bixby brought out sadness in all of us.

Bixby's new handler, Isabelle, seemed kind and gentle. Isabelle confirmed our initial assumptions by saying Bixby slept on the bed beside her. If the person leading Bixby had a mean disposition, the devastated reactions would be difficult to manage.

Summer Fun

I didn't realize just how long my convocation would be. Luckily my group went in the afternoon because I didn't do mornings well. The more time ticked by, the more reminiscing I could do.

*****

In March of 1985, my parents planned to install an in-ground pool in our backyard. My brothers and I geared up for an unforgettable summer in our own pool. Chad and Will daydreamed of doing a cannonball in our backyard.

Construction began in May of 1985. At long last the back-hoe that was digging the pool began sculpting the shallow end where the steps would eventually go. The workers used the yellow Caterpillar machine to dig the deep end.

The machine made a chugging sound. Connor Van, a two year old, who lived in a neighbouring home on the crescent, had toddled over to see the construction in action. Landon, Connor's little brother, peered around the corner of the garage to see the machines at work. Once Mrs. Van saw Chad corralled all of the little people, she went back to her Adirondack chair under the shade of a maple tree on her front lawn. Chad kept the toddlers safe and out of the way of the construction team

.As a two and a half year old, I peed before I entered the pool and the same afterwards. A great incentive to toilet train. I was ready to give up diapers, so I had no trouble.

*****

My parents printed some flyers containing information regarding swimming lessons in our pool. My brothers distributed them to families in our neighbourhood and we waited for a response.

Swimming lessons in the McIntyre' pool.
Taught by a Red Cross Certified Instructor
$20.00 per child.
*Each toddler must have adult accompaniment with them in the water.
Our older boys will be available if needed.
Classes start next Monday at 10:00AM.
We hope to see you there.
Please
R.S.V.P.

The neighbourhood parents and children loved the swimming classes and we reached capacity in no time. Everyone had pool fever in our neighbourhood. People craved a pool in their own backyard. We heated the water by covering the pool in a solar blanket. The more the sun shined, the warmer the water temperature became.

By the time July came around, we swam every day. From mid-morning to early evening we either bathed in the sun poolside or relaxed in the water. My skin turned a light brown.

*****

Fast forward to November of 1987; I was almost 5 years old. I was growing up. My Mom read an ad swimming lessons at the registration at the local YMCA. She cut out the notice from the paper and pinned the form to our cork board. Their water was warm, so I nodded.

During March of 1988, I completed my level 2 badge for swimming. I liked swimming lessons, but the deep end frightened me. I preferred to play in the shallow end of our pool, where I could decompress and float about. I didn't have to sign up for another session of swimming lessons if I wasn't keen. My mother felt unsure of how to proceed.

*****

Most kindergarten children freely used either hand to print or draw. Colouring caused my fingers to cramp up, so I would switch hands and keep right on doing my art project. Why stop doing crafts when a perfectly good hand was all set to tag me out? If I cut something out, I'd scissor up the page and switch hands to go up the other side. Logic said to turn the page, but I chose to use a fresh hand.

Quite a few kindergarten kids picked their dominant hand midway through the year. Time tends to sort out which hand a person would end up using. The odd problem persists and choosing a hand becomes tough.

My parents thought because I used both hands so well I might be ambidextrous. By the time grade one came, the teacher encouraged me to use my right hand to print because most of the other students used that hand. Mrs. Poulet was a sweet lady who meant well. Every time she saw me use my left hand, she'd move the pencil back to the right hand. I found the atmosphere of school to be stressful.

My parents concern grew because I should be able to associate joy with school. I was frustrated in the first grade. My Mom took out a sheet of primary lined paper and folded it in half. She printed my name and a short sentence on each of the two sides of paper. I copied the words down the left side of the page using my left hand and the same on the right side with my right hand.

When I completed the exercise, my parents stared at the words side by side. The printing done with my left hand showed a fraction better. My Mom came to the school at recess to chat with Mrs. Poulet. After seeing the sheet of words, the two women agreed I should use my left hand for most activities.

How do you teach a child left from right? Ask a teacher to find out. My mother painted my left baby finger with nail polish. When I printed I had a visual reminder.

When my class used scissors, I was usually given left-handed scissors. Oddly enough, I couldn't make the left handed scissors work. I'd wait a polite period and walk to the back of the room and quietly exchange the scissors for a right handed pair. I tired of doing the same song and dance every time we used scissors, so my parents bought me a pair of safety scissors to keep in my pencil case.

*****

When July came and school finished for the summer, I remained on cloud nine just hanging out by the pool. The pressure of school and swimming lessons fled my body. Getting used to the water and the changing space around me in the pool got increasingly strenuous.

I swam through the hoops on the shallow end floor. I stood on the diving board, steadying myself as I tossed the pool noodle on the water with a giant splashing sound. I jumped off of the diving board onto the fat yellow noodle.

In my head, I floated gracefully on the water akin to a swan. Clearly my swimming ability wouldn't get me many awards. Lifeguarding required immense focus and all of my energy concentrated on me staying above the water. My high spirits continued while in the pool, despite not being able to achieve greatness in the water.

Chad stepped up to the diving board, dove in and came up beside me in the water. What he could do in the water left me in awe of his abilities. As the years went by, the McIntyre kids still gravitated to the backyard pool.

During the summer, my hair turned green from the chlorine. Not a pretty look for me. My hairdresser at the time told my Mother to rinse my hair with vinegar or lemon juice at the end of my shower. Vinegar smelled comparable to body odor, so I opted for lemon juice. Sure enough, my hair returned to a shiny blonde, naturally, highlighted by the sun.

I went up to my room to change into a swimsuit for an evening swim and all of my bikinis hung damp in the bathroom. If you thought taking off a wet bathing suit could be difficult, try putting one on. My Mom said to wear the yellow jumper instead. The top buttoned to the bottom, so my nipples would be covered. The outfit wouldn't fit me much longer, so if the chlorine water wrecked the fabric I wouldn't ruin a cherished piece of my wardrobe.

I swam by myself while my Mom lifeguarded. If I appeared like I was in a wet t-shirt contest nobody would notice. I dipped my toe in the water and threw in a pool noodle. The water felt warmer than the air, so I walked right in. As I got wet, air flew up my jumper. The boobs of my dreams arrived, if only for a second. My mother laughed at me as I attempted to support my new found boobs. What a goofy kid.

*****

My Dad and brothers set up our tent by the fire pit for a few days each summer and we'd take turns having friends over to camp in our backyard. I camped outside with Norah and had lots of fun.

We'd roast hotdogs over the fire pit, followed by marshmallows. One marshmallow fell into the fire. I loved watching it puff up until sugar packed glop exploded deep within the fire, leaving gooey bits on some of the wood. A golden brown marshmallow tasted oh so sweet. My Mom would eat the really charred ones. I don't know whether she actually liked the burnt marshmallows, or just didn't want me to be upset I caught a marshmallow on fire.

I remember tenting out back with a few of my girlfriends. We would stumble inside in the morning to the smell of breakfast sausages and maple syrup. My friends impressed by the spread of food. I gulped a small glass of orange juice and burped. I didn't belch on purpose. Well, not that time anyways. My parents and friends tilted their heads back and laughed with me. I had a silent chuckle when something struck me funny.

*****

I was starting the third grade in September of 1990. Before the summer ended my family went to visit a farm where they had a litter of mixed breed puppies. A teacher on my Dad's staff had suggested that we all go and have a gander at the pups.

After raising Bixby to be a guide dog for a year, we didn't yearn to for a dog we had to give back at any point in time. My family desired a dog to call our own.

I gather my parents had discussed getting a puppy before driving out to the farm where the pups greeted us. We drove up the stone driveway and piled out of the van to a pen of the cutest fur babies I had ever seen.

We didn't bring a puppy to our house right then because the breeders suggested bringing her home during the daytime to allow the dog to acclimatize to us and our home. My family came back the next day to pick up our new bundle of fuzz.

The pup came home wrapped in a blanket she used on the farm, so a piece of her family carried her to her forever home. The Saturday of the Labour Day long weekend typically created stress, but we added a puppy into the mix. Poor planning on our part because we all headed back to school the following Tuesday. The boys would come home from high school at lunch to let her do her business burn off some excess energy. Thirty-five dollars for a dog of any kind pet seemed a steal.

We named our newest family member. My brothers and I tossed around ideas for names, but we couldn't agree. A neighbour came up with Lassie because she was part Collie. We all liked the idea. My Mom poured over the books about Lassie and adored each chapter despite the fact the novels depressed the reader.

*****

64

My fourth grade teacher Mrs. Jansen taught me not just academics, but skills for life. For example, her class learned a girl could do whatever she put her mind to. Some jobs stereotypically done by a man, but certainly didn't mean a girl shouldn't go into a particular field. I decided the next activity I would take a chance and participate, even if society said the hobby was pursued by mostly boys.

I ate all of my lunch and I took any leftover snacks home. Caroline Welder stood tall enough to be an adult and spent lunch in my classroom. She would constantly ask for my food. I made sure I never left alone because she scared me.

One day Caroline became overly pushy. She kept saying my family had money. I had no idea what kind of family she had, but her begging day after day grew tiresome. My parents did well for themselves and provided a beautiful home for my brothers and me. In fact, I heard my Dad talk about our family being comfortably in the middle class. Caroline thought I lied even after I told her we belonged in the middle class. Eventually Caroline was ordered to eat her lunch in a place where more supervision was provided.

*****

Auntie Leona and Uncle Ted invited me to go camping in Elora later that summer. Being a princess, I loved the creature comforts of home. I'd make camping fun. I put gender norms aside and signed up. Norah, my sister-cousin was one of my favourite past times. I didn't know a lot about camping. We would have an adventure together.

To a nine year old, waiting didn't produce fun. When August arrived I got pumped to go camping with my cousin. I wondered how long the drive to the campground would be. Norah peered out the car window on the way to the campsite.

My Auntie pointed me in the direction of the outhouse to go pee. Some people pee when they're nervous. I had the opposite problem. I clammed up and couldn't pee when I became anxious.

The outhouse smelled of number two. I gagged at the pine scented air freshener, obviously changed long ago. If I felt uncomfortable peeing in the outhouse, I could go in the woods. Not caring to argue, Auntie Leona compromised. I grabbed some toilet paper and a small bag to put the paper in when I concluded my business. I wandered into the dense woods and picked a spot to pee.

I came to a place and I prepared to pee by pulling my shorts down. I peed in among the trees like my aunt said, but it went in my underwear and shorts. Oh no. I suppose the situation could've been worse if I'd gone number two.

I didn't squat. Girls couldn't pee standing up. Girls crouched down to pee. My brothers went pee standing up, so I thought I could too. I hiccupped and calmed down.

My Auntie Leona got me cleaned up and changed into new shorts while trying to suppress her own laughter. She saved the story for my parents. How could my Dad miss telling me girls can't pee while remaining upright? The tale was destined to become a classic among our family.

On the first afternoon of our camping trip we were going to attempt white water rafting down the gorge. White water rafting could then be checked off my bucket list. I visualized the actual record of places I wanted to go and items I wished to complete at some point in the future.

I had a fabulous time camping with Norah, if you forget about me failing at peeing in the wooded area. We had pleasurable evenings around the campfire with the other families we were camping with.

When night fell, we slept in a tent by ourselves. My Auntie Leona informed me that when they checked on us before bed I had one leg in my sleeping bag and one leg on top. I slept like a starfish in my own bed, so a sleeping bag didn't differ... The night temperatures lowered a bit during the night, but not enough to worry my bare leg might get cold. My Uncle Ted found a blanket to cover me up before the lights went out.

*****

I joined the neighbourhood full of boys. Maybe that's why I didn't know girls couldn't pee standing up. I played baseball, road hockey, and everything in between alongside kids from our street and the surrounding area.

I never minded being the only girl. I volunteered to be in net when the kids participated in a game of road hockey, so I avoided getting sweaty. I found a point of reference and the point of view constantly changed.

*****

My brothers babysat me on the rare occasion my parents both left the house. On one particular summer afternoon our parents went to the home renovation center. The boys and I goofed around in the living room.

Chad brought a plate of green grapes from the kitchen for us to snack on. Will wondered how many grapes he could fit in his mouth and still speak. I lost count at fifteen. I followed their lead, so one by one the grapes went in my mouth. I attempted to say the word truck. The directions seemed simple enough, but with a full mouth what came out resembled a swear word. The boys' jaws dropped. Of course they knew what the word truck sounded like.

The grapes burst and my face wrinkled from the sour taste. Somebody threatened to tell our parents jokingly. By I swallowed the last grape my t-shirt covered in a mixture of drool and tears. After we all promised not to breathe a word to anyone the afternoon went merrily along.

My brothers taught me a lot, some good, some bad. Every minute spent at my brothers' side was entertaining to say the least. I put my hand in the ring whenever possible.

*****

Norah and I went for a sleepover at Grandma McIntyre' house. Our Grandma always provided fun for the two of us. Whether we walked to the post office or stopped off at a nearby park, we had a relaxing getaway.

We took our bags up to the girl's room and returned to the kitchen to assist Grandma in baking cookies. We wore cute aprons, so we didn't mess up our nice clothes.

Grandma made the ginger snap cookie dough before our arrival, so it had time to firm up in the fridge. She knew the exciting part for us was forming the cookies.

We rolled a piece of dough into a ball a bit larger than a quarter. Next we rotated the balls in sugar and placed them three fingers apart from one another to allow the cookies to spread as they baked. Before the cookies went into the oven Grandma pressed each cookie using a fork. In my mind, Grandma was stamping each cookie with her signature love.

While the cookies baked, Norah and I peeked inside through the glass door to see the sugar sparkle. After a minute we started to clean up the mess from our afternoon activities.

Grandma leaned inside the fridge and pulled out a container of homemade chunky apple sauce for us to snack on. The lid released the aroma of cinnamon and apples. I tasted the first spoonful and was not disappointed.

I didn't have many sleepovers at Grandma Porter's house, probably because we saw her on most Sundays for dinner. I do remember lying next to my Grandmother in her big bed. She snored quite loudly. We stayed up to tune into the late night talk show. I couldn't believe her small television didn't have a remote and the picture displayed in black and white.

*****

During the winter of 1993, my parents brought up Rocky Ridge Horseback Riding Christian Camp. If I opted to attend the camp, I'd be sleeping in a cabin and learning about horseback riding for a whole week. My mother and I continued to set the table for Sunday dinner.

I'd be finishing sixth grade, by the point the summer camp week grew close. I'd be roughly the same age as Will camped at the same establishment.

Would I be by myself, or with people I didn't know? I drew comfort from the fact my cousin Norah would go with me and sleep in the same cabin.

Chad and Will went to Rocky Ridge. Reese Able and Tyson Ransom and a bunch of neighbourhood kids all ended up in one cabin. Campers took a little slice of the Rocky Ridge experience home. Opportunities to explore activities such as: horseback riding, swimming, tennis, and basketball happened on a daily basis. Will reminisced.

I convinced myself I'd make fond memories to last a lifetime. Will said I could wear my pyjamas to breakfast. I'd never been away from home except for overnight at Grandma's or Norah's house. I would be alright as long as Norah came with me. Being the older cousin meant I had to console Norah if she missed home.

School let out for the summer. I helped to prepare my toiletries for camp. My mother labeled my camp gear with my name. Auntie Leona made some labels that said Norah Fairmont, so our clothing stayed in our hands. My mother read the camp newsletter. Norah and I signed up for a Walt Disney themed week in late July.

Grandma Porter had taken me for a trail ride at a farm on the outskirts of Niagara years ago. I worried about riding a horse because the last time I road on a horse, I had a dizzy spell. A brief hug from my Mom calmed my fears. She grinned and I believed camp would be a great experience.

My family hadn't been to church since I cried during the service. What if I didn't pray right? Could a person pray wrong? My concerns dripped from my mouth like melting ice-cream.

My mother reassured me the staff showed campers what to do. Norah would be by my side, so we could lean on one another. My Mom offered a slight smile, hoping to decrease my anxiety. Norah frequented church more than me, so she'd be aware of the expectations.

The end of July came around slowly. I cheered when the date camp began arrived. The Rocky Ridge Ranch directions said the drive took an hour from Niagara Falls. My Dad stared at the route, marked with a yellow highlighter.

I noticed the camp nestled in the woods off the beaten path. My Dad drove along a gravel road toward the entrance. I saw the cabins and the horse corral next to a large red barn.

I looked at the log cabin with the words "Mess Hall" carved into a yellow oval sign above the main entrance. The campers and staff ate their meals at the mess hall.

I saw a swimming pool up on a hill. Riding a horse stirred up some apprehension. I'd be able to push through my fear and learn all aspects of farm life. I gathered the large white building beyond the barn to be the chapel. I took in all of the visual stimuli around me.

Paige Oaken led my cabin for the week. She hailed from Halifax, Nova Scotia. Paige instructed her campers to grab a bunk and organize our things.

We started by introducing ourselves and telling everyone where we lived. Tonya's family grew up outside of Stratford. Ramona resided in the university town of London. Isabella (or Bella for short) dwelled in Kitchener. Chelsea stayed from Orangeville. My cabin mates all came from Ontario except for our counsellor.

Before we headed to the chapel for the welcome meeting, Paige went over a few rules. "The washrooms and showers are just up the hill, to the right of our cabin as we exit the door. The washrooms have spiders, but we must shower. We don't want anyone to stink up our cabin." She wrinkled her nose as her lips slowly curved upward.

The clothes any person wore to the barn, shouldn't be worn anywhere else. The outfit would contain an odor of the horses.

Each camper chose an outfit to wear to the dining hall and church services. A t-shirt and khaki pants suited both places. No one expected the kids to dress-up in skirts and blouses.

I guess wearing my pyjamas to breakfast wouldn't fly. I brought extra clothes for mealtime to be on the safe side.

Every camper's parents put money aside for their child to spend at the tuck shop each night after the chapel service. The tuck shop sold chips, popsicles, ice cream bars, and a wide variety of penny candies. Counsellors coached their kids to choose wisely because the tuck shop money had to last all week.

Jeb and his wife Chelsea welcomed everyone to Rocky Ridge Ranch.

Dear Lord,
May you watch over all of our campers now and always. Let this be a week filled with joy for everyone. Bless us O Lord.
Amen.

Lucky for me, a laminated page on the back of each pew included the words to the short opening remarks.

Chelsea prayed we all had a wonderful week at camp. The staff trusted the students listened to their respective counsellors. The first two rows, paved the way to the dining hall for lunch and the other rows followed in an orderly fashion.

After my cabin ate, we all put on our barn clothes so we could meet our horse for the week. Paige clapped her hands, rounding up her campers.

Paige glanced at me and Norah thinking we might be related. She saw a family resemblance. I delighted someone thought Norah and I looked alike. Norah was adopted, but we maintained comparable hair styles and height. Blood doesn't necessarily make a family; close relationships do. I would forever be grateful to Norah's birth family for bringing us together. Life wouldn't have been the same without my best friend.

A horse named Paul Bee was mine for the week. Norah rode Chestnut. Jeb matched all of the campers to a horse. We had to learn take care of the horses and their equipment before we could ride them. I finished up with my horse and waited quietly for my counsellor.

We followed Paige to our cabin to change out of our barn clothes. Normally we would have free time to play basketball, swim, or play miniature golf, but since our first day started at noon, we only had a short time before dinner. We played a game to get to know each other.

*****

The kitchen prepared a smaller meal for dinner and a bigger meal at lunchtime because we burned a lot of energy during the day. The hot turkey sandwiches dribbled onto my plate. Gravy trickled from the corners of my mouth, but nobody minded the mess.

When we polished off our supper, we waited for our cabin leader and skipped to the chapel. The benches felt awfully hard. My joints stiffened due to the active day, so I sat down.

After a brief delay, I placed my order at the tuck shop. I ordered five hot lips and five fuzzy peaches and spent under a dollar. Norah had a bag of ketchup chips and a cream soda.

Paige sat on her bed next to her bag of plain chips. We filled our bellies with snacks. Paige started the nightly Bible study. I silently prayed for spiritual guidance.

Dear Lord,
I'm sorry that I haven't kept in touch better over the years. Please don't have
Paige ask me any question that I can't handle.
Many thanks,
Megan McIntyre

I saw a pattern. If a sentence opened with 'Dear Lord', the following statements usually constituted a prayer. If a thought concluded in 'Amen', the prior statements involved a prayer of some sort.

Paige had several passages marked with bright coloured highlighters and mini sticky notes. She asked, "How do we know God is around us?"

Paige blinked up at me on the top bunk. My mouth was dry, but I gave an answer anyway.

I whispered, "The great events happening all around us are His doing. God also helps us to see the good even in a bad situation." I anticipated the bible study questions getting easier as I got used to the biblical interactions.

I had no trouble falling asleep the first night of camp. I envisioned being on horseback.

*****

Hop on up. Jeb was right behind me as I mounted my horse. I went on out to the corral and started a slow ride around the ring. Butterflies danced in my tummy, creating a nauseous feeling in my throat. I told myself that everyone had the same sensation. I got over my panicky mode and I took control of my horse. I snapped a photo in my head.

After two full days at camp, we signed up for a race on rodeo day. Paige read us the details of each race. I chose to do the cracker race. I trotted down the corral to a staff member, who gave me five crackers. I ate as fast as I could and said Rocky Ridge Ranch without spraying food bits everywhere. Norah decided on the same race as me.

When parents came to pick us up on Saturday afternoon, the campers showed off their abilities in a rodeo. Paige folded the sign-up sheet and slid the paper into a manila envelope. I got to ride Maple for the cracker race and Norah would be riding Chestnut for the rodeo.

And the first heat of the rodeo commenced.

I scoffed my boots in disgust. Maple went a few feet and stopped to take the world's longest poop in the middle of my race. My Uncle Ted thought the crap was a personal best for my horse. My Auntie Leona swatted his arm.

I hugged my parents simultaneously. My Uncle Ted videotaped the whole race, so now we could watch my horse poo for eternity. My mother wiped her lipstick off my cheek using spit and a finger. My parents missed me.

I crossed my arms and turned to watch the other races. A few races after mine, Maple won the bubble gum race. I pouted and kicked some more dirt. Of course Maple won, he had the shit of a lifetime during my race.

I had a fabulous week at camp, but I was glad to see my parents.

Norah and I flipped through our camp photos and laughed at our wardrobe choices. Our high wasted shorts and floral prints hadn't come into style yet. We both giggled every time we watched the camp video.

*****

At eleven years old, I was completing the sixth grade. Softball registration came on the second weekend of February. I asked myself if playing ball in the summer made me happy. I didn't know yet what to do. I wished I could play t-ball again. Everybody batted every inning and the game ended in a tie.

I decided to sign on for another year of softball. I joyfully thought of playing baseball under the lights at the local ballpark. Travel baseball wasn't attainable for me, but I made the most of the sport.

The long weekend in May marked my first baseball practice of the season. The youngest player on my team happened to be me. My frame weighed in at just below sixty-five pounds, so I also received the petite player award.

I observed the Toronto Blue Jays on the television. I wished I could play second base like Roberto Alomar. He played the game with such ease. I was not exactly a star baseball player and the dents in our garage door to proved it.

In June, I'd had a few practices and a couple of games. I didn't enjoy baseball as much. My coach acted like we played on an elite travel team instead of a house league one. She annoyed me.

I asked my Dad to throw the ball around after dinner. He grinned at me. Throwing the ball around with my Dad was something we could do together. My Dad coached Chad's travel baseball team. He had a much nicer way of dealing with the players than my coach did. I wished my Dad could be my coach.

Even though I'm left-handed, I played baseball right handed. When I played road hockey, I shot the puck right handed. I studied my brothers' and used their old hockey sticks. I was never going to be a hockey star.

My Dad's arm began getting sore, but he didn't stop for fear of disappointing me.

Connor called from his front lawn, already dressed in his Hawaiian swimsuit. He hollered at me to come swimming at his house. My Dad winked and I went to change into my tankini.

*****

During July, I spent a lot of time in the pool. I had a tan line from my two piece bathing suit to prove it. I liked my skin to turn golden brown in the warmer months. By the end of the winter, I returned to my natural pasty white colouring.

I thought the late summer night would be perfect weather to start a fire pit. I wrapped in a towel shivering, fresh from the neighbour's pool.

My Dad grabbed a flashlight and the barbeque lighter and headed out the sliding door to the backyard to set the chairs up and gather the wood for the fire.

My Mom cupped her hands around her coffee mug and sat on a light green lawn chair by the fire pit. We retreated to the backyard during the summer months.

If I intended on having a cottage, I had to marry into a family with a vacation home on a lake. Our lot was just less than half an acre, with a large deck, mature maple trees, a pool and a campfire. We had the amenities and atmosphere of a northern property.

Camping in our backyard allowed me to have all of the comforts of home close by if I required. I could pee indoors when the campsite was steps away from a bathroom. My lips went from a slight frown to a full blown smile. I learned the hard way that girls couldn't pee standing up.

High School Life

I patiently waited for my name to be called. I sat perfectly still in the front of the Brock University gymnasium. Soon I would be rolled across the stage so I could receive my degree in psychology. The speaker went on and on. How was her mouth not as dry as the Mojave Desert? I wasn't speaking to anyone and I was thirsty.

*****

Back in August of 1996, I prepared to start high school, an exciting time for teenagers. I would be going from a big fish in a little pond, to a small fish in a big pond. I was in the middle of a scary transition in life. Once I found my place among the big fish, I hoped for less stress in my life.

I had my first day of high school in September. My friends and I decided to walk to school together, at least in the beginning of the school year. I dreaded the walk to school. Every textbook seemed to add a lot of weight to my backpack.

I wasn't fourteen years old yet. Signs of fall crept around us. My friends and I broke off and made new connections. They didn't eat lunch together or hang out on weekends. What should I have done? Unfortunately, friends do go in different directions in high school. I refused to eat alone or at the misfit table. I'd made a few friends in my classes; I decided I would join one of them at their lunch table. I'd make some new friends in no time.

I stood beside Olivia Mason's locker as she retrieved her lunch from her school bag. She didn't mind if I ate at her lunch table. Basically my friends from elementary school had elected to hang out with other people. What a bummer?

Olivia had been through similar events with some of her middle school friends. There wasn't a defining moment per se. Her friends stopped calling in much the same way my friendships petered out.

*****

November arrived quickly. I turned fourteen and had established routines in high school. I didn't quite "love" every situation, but I was comfortable with my daily schedule.

My first class of the day was music. We learned to play an instrument in an ensemble. I started out trying to get a note out of the flute because the case didn't weigh much. No way would I be able to lug home a tuba or a French horn.

I couldn't get a sound out of the flute. I persisted in asking any musical person I knew for assistance. Norah was a flautist in the Burlington Teen Tour Band and her advice still had me silent.

I had to face the music; I would have to pick a new instrument. The clarinet was the next smallest woodwind instrument, but it didn't seem any simpler than the flute. I muddled through the classes and my practices sounded like I was torturing a cat. If I continued with music, I'd buy my family ear plugs.

The class had a chamber concert at the end of the term. Right before we walked out to a sea of proud parents, my reed broke. I smoothed it out as best I could, but I worried the audience would discover how little musical ability I had.

When the music portion of the semester ended, art class began.

"I hope you love art." My music teacher saw how hard I tried and a good part of my grade came in part due to my effort. I appreciated his sentiments, and at some point I saw the humour in my music teacher's words.

*****

Art class was a lot more joyful for me than struggling to make a note out of any instrument in the music room. My art teacher, Mr. Jibbers, was eccentric in his mannerisms.

One morning he instructed the class to bring a chair and form a circle. We ended up with a misshapen oval. Mr. Jibbers started his lesson by adding an empty chair for a guest named Roy G. Biv. The initials sunk in and my classmates and I understood that Roy was an acronym for the colours on the colour wheel.

Dean Sensor arrived to our art class late, so he took a seat in the empty chair. Mr. Jibbers cried out when Dean sat on Roy G. Biv. Dean's confusion evident due to the creases in his forehead.

*****

About two months into the ninth grade, students went to work with a parent. My Dad retired when I ended the eighth grade, so I couldn't go to work join him in leisure activities.

My Mom taught first grade, so I thought I'd get a sense for teaching young children. I babysat young kids, but I figured teaching would be harder. I'd have to get used to the large number of six year olds.

My Mom informed me that Mrs. Sensor's son would be coming to Take Your Kid to Work Day with his mother. Dean appeared to have a wicked sense of humor. I'd have a pleasurable day regardless, but being near Dean ensured I'd be in stitches at least once before the day wrapped up.

I spent the morning in my Mom's classroom. At lunch time, Mrs. Sensor, Dean, my Mom and I went to a sub shop up the road from the elementary school.

After the kids returned to start the afternoon, I followed the class to the gym with Mrs. Sensor and Dean. Mrs. Sensor had a mini gymnastics circuit set up around the perimeter of the gym. Dean and I assisted at the somersault station. As the kids did a somersault, they moved to the next station. We clapped and cheered even for the children who did a poor attempt of a somersault. Dean looked at me and mouthed "really", as children flowed through our station. Who can't do simple gymnastics?

When recess came Dean and I accompanied our mothers on yard duty. I noticed one older child was an extremely close talker. Mrs. Sensor backed up from the kid. Dean's face showed his emotions. He readied himself to step in, but Mrs. Sensor indicated she could handle the tall boy. The boy towered over her, but she redirected him. He invaded her personal space and that didn't sit well with Dean.

*****

Friday night Olivia invited me to watch a movie at her house. She slouched against the row of purple lockers. That sounded like a good idea to me. I carefully replaced the cap on the lip balm and smacked my lips together. The lip gloss was for Caleb Finnigan. He happened to have the locker next to me and I had a crush on him. Olivia said to bring my Mom, if she was free. Her Mom would make tea and they could chat.

My mother, Rose, squinted as her muddy brown eyes adjusted to the soft interior lighting. After Josie Mason introduced herself, she brushed her light brown bangs to the side.

Rose and Josie were both only children. Their fathers both bus drivers for neighbouring cities. The two ladies had lots in common. Josie poured the boiling water into her brown tea pot.

My maternal grandfather, Aaron Porter, was a union rep for St. Catharines. He passed away long before I could meet him.

Josie's father was Henry Routers, but everyone (including the girls) called him Hop. Pepsi was on sale at the other end of town and the sale started tonight, so Hop would drop off some pop on his way home. Hop was always ready for a good bargain, even when he had to drive miles out of his way to save a few dollars. The storm door opened and Hop hollered for Josie in a deep crackly voice.

He began to stack the pop at the side of the hall. Olivia would bring the cases downstairs to the bar. Josie walked to the hallway, motioning for my Mother to follow.

Josie introduced Rose and explained the connection to her Dad. Hop was about six feet tall, a large frame, a thatch of snow white hair and the look of a sweet grandfather. My Mom explained her father was the late Aaron Porter. He stretched over six feet in height, a slender man with light hair and a kind heart.

Hop said he knew Zip Porter from the union meetings and he devoted his life to his wife and daughter. Hop's face lit up, taking him back to his days as a bus driver.

Nobody knows why they called my Grandpa Zip. The nickname was passed down from his father. What I wouldn't give to be able talk with either of my grandfathers. If I couldn't connect with my own grandfathers, I had Hop in my life. Anybody who remembered my Grandpa, I considered to be a piece of my Grandpa Porter.

Liv handed me a soda and I slid a straw into it. I took a long gulp and continued watching the movie. Something struck me as funny and I opened my mouth to laugh and out came a huge burp followed by a few baby burps. Olivia, her sister Kate and I kept the giggly mood going for the rest of the evening. Once I had belched, the proverbial cat couldn't be shoved back in the bag.

*****

I sat in my sociology class, minding my own business, when I saw Ian Payer motion to another girl to pull his finger. I knew that predicted a fart. I had brothers, while my classmate had two sisters. Girls who didn't have brothers had much to learn, but I never tired of watching ladies get educated in the art of boys.

Ian's family had four boys and no girls. Surely at times their family room smelled like farts and old gym socks. Until one of the boys had a girl over, then the room saturated with cologne.

*****

Eleventh grade high school went well. The social aspect carried on during lunch, after school, and on weekends. The best part of being a teenager had nothing to do with academics. Whether I watched a movie with Olivia or order dinner at Tyler's house, believed maintaining friendships an important part of my education. My self-esteem and confidence hit an all-time high.

Olivia and I registered for a cooking class in high school. Dean Sensor made the class list, so at the very least we would have fun.

My group read a recipe in the kitchen. The washing machine had an unbalanced load, so Dean plopped down on top lid and rode in into the sunset like a cowboy. I couldn't wait until the shit hit the fan on that one.

*****

Olivia said I had to meet one of her lifeguard friends, Jonah Fletcher. He appeared rather attractive in a rugged way from the pictures I had seen. Olivia flushed at the mention of Jonah's name.

Jonah did his lifeguard recertification the weekend before and Olivia recognized him from assisting in the city swim lessons the previous year. I would volunteer to practice CPR on Jonah.

The month of May brought sunshine. The grass returned to a vibrant green. The flowers started to bloom. Mother Nature had awakened from a long winter nap.

Every year a dance competition in the spring made the way to a high school auditorium. Ballet dancers envied the arches in my feet. Dancers' balanced easily. Tap, jazz, hip-hop, acrobatics and lyrical ballet all left me clueless. From recitals and dance contest gave me the ability to tell which groups performed better than others. Olivia and Kate danced in several different numbers I found entertaining.

When Olivia came out to the auditorium to talk to me, a hot guy stepped forward to greet her. Jonah Fletcher shook my hand. Liv knew him from city lifeguarding. He came to see his girlfriend dance, but semantics didn't matter. Jonah wore a wrinkled t-shirt, but he seemed to make the shirt work.

I reluctantly pulled my eyes away from Jonah to meet his friend Boyd Ryerson. The two boys stood at the top of the auditorium looking casual. Boyd had a goofiness about him, which made him attractive.

*****

Hi Megan,
I have a lifeguard meet and greet next week, so I'll try and set something up with Jonah and his friends after our finals are over.
Olivia

At the beginning of June, Olivia turned seventeen. When Olivia and I stopped studying for our final exams, we busily made summer plans. Even though most of our friends worked for the summer jobs, I sensed greater freedom because everyone had our own money to spend.

I held my backpack over one shoulder as Liv and I waited for my mother to pick us up from our last exam. Summer heat and humidity, made perfect swimming conditions.

Hi Megan.
Jonah's friends, Boyd and Cooper Hadley are meeting us at the mini golf downtown on Friday around 7. Boyd collected Jonah at work a few days ago. He's a handful from what I can gather. The other guys I don't know.
It's a great way to start off our summer.
Olivia

I talked to my parents about where I was going and in which car. I figured concerned parents of a teenage daughter deserved to have all of the information. They didn't give me a curfew and I didn't drive.

"Some of the guys Liv and I are meeting are strikingly handsome. I won't be engaging in any activity that will affect me in nine months." Honesty worked the best policy when dealing with my parents. Communication between my parents and I was open and they respected me for my candor.

I'd only spent a little time in the company of Jonah, but I trusted him in all ways.

Mini-putt created an interesting environment. Olivia parked her parent's minivan. Jonah was still in his bathing suit, but added a hoodie over his lifeguard singlet and he pulled it off so well. I wished I could not let what other people think of me dictate what I clothed myself in.

Jonah spotted us and flashed his perfect smile, showing his dimples. He wrapped his arms around me and I breathed in the scent of his deodorant and a strong scented fabric softener. Jonah blew his curly mop of golden brown hair off his face.

He lifted Olivia off the ground and intense happiness showed upon her cheeks. When Olivia was on the lifeguard chair and the other guards called her, she didn't pay attention to any of them. The pool often had two or three swimmers named Olivia at any given moment. When her name is called, she doesn't figure anyone is referring to her. The nickname Liv was born out of necessity.

Boyd Ryerson caught up to Jonah and yelled "Livy and Megannnnnnn." apparently I had a pet name. Boyd looked at me, an evil grin on graced his face and a sparkle in his eyes. I didn't mind being referred to as "Megannnnnnn". Clearly Jonah chatted about Liv and me to his friends.

Cooper Hadley held out two shiny green golf balls and offered to let me touch his balls. His manner made me laugh. The golf balls matched his hair. Cooper somehow made neon green hair look cute.

Cooper dyed his hair for school spirit week, which coincidently corresponded to the day of graduation pictures. His mother wasn't too pleased his last minute choice to change his natural hair colour. Everyone else adored his new edgy style.

I formed a team next to on Cooper. He sported a partially zipped horizontal striped hoodie. Cooper's clothing matched nothing he dressed in and yet he still looked hot and well put together.

Olivia and I fretted which shirt to wear an hour before coming to the mini-putt. We checked out our lip gloss in the visor mirror before getting out of the minivan. The guys put little to no effort into their outfits and managed to look beyond gorgeous. Life wasn't fair.

I had played mini-putt a lot in Myrtle Beach, but Cooper wasn't aware of that fact. Cooper grabbed my putter and stood behind me to demonstrate his putting skills. He wrapped his arms around me and took a practice swing. Jonah pointed out my lipstick. He wondered if I planned on wearing the wine coloured lip stain off. I hadn't thought far ahead to be frank.

I got a hole in one. I beamed a smile, showing off my perfectly straight teeth that years of orthodontist visits made possible. My bucked teeth gradually disappeared as my braces altered my jaw line. I high fived Cooper and slowly grabbed my ball.

Jonah planned for us to meet everyone at his house on Friday around six o'clock. Olivia anticipated the event all week. "That'll be fun", I pumped my hands in the air.

Liv and I began hanging out with Carly Newl during the previous school year. Carly had been craving a Dairy Queen Blizzard that day. A new cotton candy menu item made my mouth water.

Olivia thought she could borrow her parents' car. I could never have enough of Dairy Queen, so I fetched my wallet. The sky was alight with orange and pink stripes. I swung my legs over the cherry red picnic table and dug in. The sugary goodness coated my pearly whites.

When Carly neared the end of her Blizzard she searched for her next endeavor. She peeked at Olivia and me above her phone. Liv and I worked early the following morning, so we'd probably head home after we finished our ice cream. We might stop to get a coffee, but nothing more.

Carly had an older cousin who came and got her up at the ice cream shop because Olivia and I planned to turn in early. Carly had slept in on her day off from a restaurant hostess position, so she had energy to burn off.

The iced cappuccino tasted creamy. I took a long sip of my drink, sitting on my front porch. Jonah had brought refreshments to the pool one day, so Liv encouraged me to try the cold treat. Olivia and I observed the neighbourhood kids soaking up the last light of the summer evening on the crescent.

Jonah emailed Liv a couple days later.

Livy.....
Do you want to go to a movie with a few of my friends? You and Megan can be in charge of what show see. Boyd, Danny Sage, and Cooper are coming too.
We'll meet you at the theatre in an hour.
Please come. We'll have a blast.
Jonah

Since I didn't drive, Olivia's car would be in my driveway in ten minutes. My eyes widened as I glanced at the clothes in my overstuffed closet. I informed my mother of my whereabouts for the evening.

I grabbed a pink hoodie and put it on over a white t-shirt and dark denim capris. I slipped on a pair of black strappy sandals and hung my charcoal coloured purse across my body. The hoodie matched my lips perfectly.

My mother lifted her reading glasses and set down her Nora Roberts novel on the coffee table. She told me I could find money in the side of her purse. I got paid on the previous Friday, so I had money in the bank and some cash from my last visit to the ATM.

I greeted Olivia, sliding awkwardly into the front seat of her gold Grand Am. I thought we should see Bring it On. After all, they said we could choose the movie.

The guys might not go for a show about cheerleading, but we felt compelled to proceed with our preference. Carly ran errands with her sister and would get dropped off at the theatre. I was glad she'd started to come out of her shell with Olivia and me.

"Bring it On." reported to be a girly movie. To my surprise, Jonah got tickets to Livy and Megan's choice. I stared at the guys and until hands raised up in defeat. I counted on some push back for a perceived lame movie option. The dancing cheerleader movie won out and we got some popcorn at the concession stand.

I wondered, "Who's that girl with Jonah?" I had confusion on my face.

Fiona Taylor was Jonah's girlfriend. Livy's shoulders shrugged. She's in the twelfth grade at our school and she's a lifeguard at Olivia's pool. I didn't know he had a girlfriend.

Fiona introduced herself. She knew all about me; while I had heard nothing regarding her. She went to Maple Street Public Elementary School, where my Mom taught primary grades.

Boyd interrupted our brief conversation like only he could do. Fiona's nickname was Fee Fee.

Carly met the guys for the first time. I realized Carly's eyes lingered on Boyd. Uh-oh.

Once the movie launched, the boys got restless. They could only stand so much dancing and cheerleading. Jonah and Cooper left to check out what was playing in the other theatres.

After the show ended, everyone craved fast food. Cooper thought a Wendy's stayed open late not far from the theatre. He ran his hand through his spiky blonde hair and highlighter yellow tips.

Eww. I pointed towards Boyd and Carly, who were lip locked. Since nobody was taken with the movie Olivia and I chose, we wouldn't be banned from selecting an activity anytime soon.

Boyd waited to see what the student council president had to say. He poked fun at Jonah's high profile status in everything he did. Jonah had the teacher stare down cold.

Jonah decided he was riding with Livy and me. Of course he hollered shot gun before I did. He ran past me and Liv on a bench near the exit.

I didn't know Jonah was student council president. Jonah turned to me in the back seat. He was anything, but stuck-up. Even people who tried not to like the guy ended up being his friend. Jonah was the kind of person who caused girls to fumble and lose their words.

"Mommy and Daddy were talking; we'll be at the restaurant soon." Jonah rubbed his smooth jaw line. Jonah was hot, intelligent, athletic and a charming personality to boot.

Jonah and his friends became part of my social circle. I got the impression Carly didn't always think the group was entertaining. She Boyd dated, but not all of the time. It depended on what Carly felt like doing, as to whether she'd be agreeable to whatever we proposed. We all understood not everyone would be up for every outing.

*****

Hi Guys.
Movie night at my house tonight. I think the lifeguards are finished work at 8 PM, so any time after that is fine by me.
By now everyone knows that I like to snack, so come ready to eat.
Megan xo

I sent out a group text message to the usual suspects and figured we'd have an interesting evening no matter which combination of my friends knocked on my front door.

Carly and Boyd had plans, but they'd try and come over at some point. Jonah wrote that he'd come after work and he'd bring Olivia.

My Dad restocked the bar fridge, so we had several different kinds of pop chilling. We had the movie channels, or some movies in a basket beside the television. I flopped my tired self on the corner couch beside Jonah.

Moments later, Boyd and Carly arrived. They had grabbed a bite to eat before joining us. Boyd held Carly's hand and proudly kissed her on the cheek.

Jonah pulled up the guide to see what television had to offer. The sex channel appeared. He fixed his eyes on me. Jonah was delighted to watch me squirm as he tuned in to see the making of vibrators.

We got all the channels because my brother worked for the satellite company and he lived in our family home. I pleaded with my friends to believe me.

Boyd gawked at the television screen and then back at me in sheer disbelief, as if he'd never seen a dirty magazine, much less a porn flick.

I admitted that I'd flipped the channel on before just to see what type of shows the station aired. I watched my friends for their reaction. I was sure the guys had seen dirty flicks before. Nobody confessed to the truth because they enjoyed seeing me blush and attempt to explain why my family subscribed to the sex channel.

The guys figured I must be sexually active. If they only knew I'd never had sex before. Shit. My face turned brick red. My new nickname was MacDaddy. Jonah aimed to keep a straight face, but failed.

Livy and I had multiple monikers and the guys had none for Carly. She wished to be included by the guys. I understood her reasoning. I was also aware you couldn't force someone to provide you a new handle.

Boyd would answer to Boydy, Ry, and Sonny. Cooper Hadley was referred to as Coop, Coo-Coo, and Haddy. Jonah got called Fletch, Jay, Joe, or Joey. Boyd also called Jonah a King Debater because he was captain of the debate team. I made a mental note to never start an argument with Jonah because I likely wouldn't win.

Carly flipped her curly hair behind her ears. Jonah suggested Car, but she didn't approve. Carly protested, while Boyd remained oblivious to the power struggle happening between his new girlfriend and his long time best friend.

Carly straightened up to go home. She looked at Olivia for help. Liv got a ride from Jonah, so she was of no help. Carly elbowed Boyd in the ribs. He peeled his eyes off of the sex channel and got up to leave.

Jonah asked if Carly was always frustrating. She could be kind if you gave her a chance. Carly liked to have a backup plan. If what we suggested wasn't an activity she enjoyed, then she'd stay home. If she received a better offer, she'd change her plans. We understood things come up now and then.

I curved my lips upward in honesty, as I raised my head up. Jonah tickled Olivia until she laughed out loud. I kept tabs on the making of vibrators on the sex channel. Jonah gently put his arm around me and lightly squeezed. I sensed I would be safe whenever he was around.

My parents thought Jonah was an all-around good guy. Boyd's loud nature could be off putting.

*****

When August of 1999 flew into town, the days got cooler. Olivia and I spent a lot of our free time with the group of guys we had become close to. In September the girls would return to one of the high schools in the city and the boys would go to another public high school at the other end of Niagara Falls.

Jonah's number showed up on Olivia's cell phone as she and I browsed the video rental store. Carly was in a different section of the store. I encouraged Olivia to hit talk. My slight frame stiffened while eavesdropping on their conversation.

Jonah suggested we bring the movie to his house. It would take us roughly twenty minutes to pick a movie and drive to Jonah's house.

Carly turned down the aisle of new releases to meet up and see what we had found. Olivia pressed the end button on her phone and mentioned to Carly about the change of plans.

I was happy to go to Jonah's house, knowing my parents would be okay with the different setting for our movie watching. Carly grew angry at Olivia and me for skipping our girls' night. We dropped Carly at her house on the way to Jonah's house.

In Carly's eyes, we had chosen Jonah over her. He phoned out of the blue and we came running. Carly crossed her arms in a major league pout. I sort of felt badly. But the fact Carly had bailed on us to do other pursuits than once made our choice sit better.

*****

During our Christmas holidays the boys gave Liv and I chocolate penises. Mine was a large white chocolate penis complete with balls. Liv got a milk chocolate penis on a stick.

We laughed and I shoved my chocolate to the back of my desk drawer. I promptly forgot about the chocolate.

When the next Valentine's Day arrived I was bitter I didn't have a boyfriend. I decided I'd bite the tip off of my chocolate penis off and eat it. As luck would have it, the chocolate didn't taste very good. I crammed the chocolate back in the clear plastic sleeve and shoved the box to the back of a drawer and promptly forgot the partially eaten candy penis existed.

Months had gone by and Chad inquired if I had any gum he could take. I told him where I kept my gum and off he went. Of course I'd forgotten the chocolate penis had been in the same drawer as my gum.

Yikes. Chad was scarred forever.

Puppy Love

People shifted in their chairs. I was getting restless at my own graduation. I tilted my neck to the left first and then the right to stretch out my tired muscles. I suspect the speeches neared the end and then the degrees would be handed out.

*****

The September prior to my fourth birthday, I started preschool. The school board in our area didn't offer junior kindergarten when I was little so I went a couple mornings a week to socialize with children of a similar age.

My Mother walked me into the gym where all of the other children had congregated. My Mom straightened my white blouse and kissed me goodbye; she'd be back to pick me up before lunch.

Connie Finlay licked her finger and wiped her lipstick off her son Tyler's face. The two women introduced themselves as Tyler and I ran off together. My Mom didn't think dropping her baby off for two hours would be so hard. She watched as the double doors swung closed and swept a tear off her cheek.

Looking at Tyler in the preschool gymnasium, my Mom knew that he would look the same way at forty years old as he presented at four years old. She thought Tyler had an old soul.

I uttered my name to a boy on a big wheel near me. His name was Tyler Finlay, although we probably didn't use our last name in preschool.

*****

A year later, I entered half day kindergarten. Ty was in my class at my big school. We participated in many of the same activities. The house centre became one of our favourite places in the classroom.

Starting half day kindergarten meant a big change for me. Going to

88

school in the morning didn't sit well with me because I would miss the arts and crafts segment on the children's television shows that interested me.

When I was a child, if you didn't see a show, you had to wait until it went into reruns. Being in the morning kindergarten class, I'd miss Mr. Dress-up. My Mom was to watch the craft while I had school. The personal video recorder had not been invented yet. How did we survive without the technology that surrounds us now?

*****

January came in with an icy start to the New Year. Indoor recesses had become a regular occurrence due to the bitterly cold weather.

My parents had planned a trip to Myrtle Beach, South Carolina over our Spring Break. Although we still had to wait two months until we would leave, we all looked forward to getting away from our daily routines.

Spring Break arrived in the middle of March. Our car was expertly packed by my Dad. I sat in the middle of the backseat with my tote bag of travel games and snacks at my feet.

I pondered who would be the first to meet someone they knew. My Dad was a school principal and well known in the community we assumed my Dad would be the winner. My brothers didn't have any friends going to Myrtle Beach over the school break.

Will rubbed my head resting on his shoulder. I just had to stay awake until we crossed the border into the United States of America. Chad raised his hand to tickle me and I squirmed in my seat. I was smiling, but we'd barely left the city limits; there was plenty of time for grumpiness to set in.

My parents told me the customs agent would inquire where I came from. The first time my Mother had done a pretend version of the situation, my response was that I was from Mommy's tummy. Oh dear.

I rubbed my sleepy eyes hoping we had reached our destination already. We had stopped in front a roadside motel. My Dad was checking to see if there was room at the Inn. I had slept for a long time. We were in Beckley, West Virginia.

I wondered if we had stumbled upon the town where Jesus was born. Perhaps I should have continued going to Sunday school. Jesus was born in Bethlehem. The Red Roof Inn wasn't around back then.

We made it to Myrtle Beach. I was happy to be on vacation with my family. My brothers took me to explore the hotel and burn off some excess energy. Will held out his hand for me to hold, so I was nestled in between the boys. They swung me back and forth down the open air corridors of our hotel. Life was fabulous.

Chad lifted me up to see over the railing of the balcony. The sandy beach and the ocean waves made music. I continued to giggle in delight, the way only a five year old can.

After we ate breakfast the next morning, we went to play a round of miniature golf. Will and Chad suggested Jungle Lagoon, just off the main highway. Will swung his arm with an imaginary golf putter.

My Dad pulled into a parking spot and we all piled out of the station wagon. The boys noticed that we were standing next to a van that was from Ontario. I grasped hold of my father's outstretched hand and walked in the direction of the ticket booth.

The mountain in the middle of the golf course seemed large to me. The people waiting for their turn to putt peered over the fence. From way above, a little voice greeted me. We all glanced up and saw Tyler and his family. I squealed as I waved up at him. I was the first person to meet someone I knew in Myrtle Beach. Go figure.

*****

The calendar read well into May. The warmer weather kept teasing us, but summer hadn't officially rolled into town. I mentioned to my Mommy one day that I liked boys. I pondered what kind of boy I'd marry when I grew up. I thought I'd like to marry a Chinese guy. My Mother knew instantly I had a crush on Spencer Born, because he was the only Asian boy in my class. He lived nearby, which was a plus, given that we had just turned five years old.

*****

By the time I reached nine years old, I had a new boy on the brain which was totally normal for a girl in my age group. Hormones hovered around my fourth grade classmates. Tyler's humor drew me into his world. I had butterflies in my stomach every time we had interactions at school.

*****

In the fall of eighth grade Ty gave me the nickname Bones because I didn't weigh much. When he referred to me as Bones my stomach began doing flips. The name from another person's mouth wouldn't be the same. Somehow my peers never used the name Bones when talking to me.

*****

I had begun the second semester of my freshman year of high school. I had lost some friends and made some new ones. My best friend Olivia Mason leaned against the lockers waiting for me to get lunch money out of my wallet.

Tyler was in my science class for the semester. I'd like to be more than friends, but if we tried to be boyfriend and girlfriend and our relationship didn't survive, I could lose him. Ty and I had fun going out for dinner or talking on the phone.

Whether we did homework, went swimming, or simply watched a movie, we never got bored of each other's company. My greatest desires involved building a life with Ty.

*****

In February of 1998 my parents announced trip to Myrtle Beach. We waited for my Spring Break to begin in March. We needed a getaway before my scheduled back surgery in June. The boys wouldn't be coming because they both had to work.

I could hardly wait for the calendar to turn the page to March. My parents and I could all use an escape from my ever growing number of doctor visits. As we left Canada, the rain peppered our windshield. We headed for sunshine, so I didn't mind leaving the drizzly weather in the rearview mirror.

Olivia and her family decided to come to Myrtle Beach and stayed at the same hotel. Tyler and his Dad opted to do a last minute father and son trip to Myrtle Beach. We elected to play a round of mini-putt at Jungle Lagoon for old time's sake.

Ty and his Dad picked me up at seven o'clock in the evening. My parents told me to invite them back to our hotel room after the game of mini-putt concluded. I paused in front of the bathroom mirror applying my pink Bonne Belle lip gloss. The flavour of strawberries and kiwi puckered my pout.

Mr. Finlay would be back to collect us later in the evening. The memories of the miniature golf course we had met at years ago flooded my mind. I took a deep breath to calm my nerves. Ty grabbed two putters and two balls and paid the teenage guy behind the counter.

We made the trek to the highest point of the golf course and froze for a minute. Ty touched the arm of my jacket in admiration. The coat belonged to my Mom, but nonetheless I appreciated the gesture. We stared at each other, but I couldn't seem to remove my gaze away from Tyler. The air fettered with pheromones surrounded the two of us. Attraction felt like a ghost between us.

Tyler and I finished the game and grabbed some soft serve ice cream at a nearby shop. I cheered inside my brain. I reveled in the cloud of happiness encircling the two of us.

Corey inquired how our golf game went. Ty got a hole in one at the highest point of the course, so he had a free pass for his next visit. I hoped we'd be back for another round someday. I could picture Ty and me bringing our kids to Myrtle Beach, retelling and embellishing the stories. Perhaps I was a tad premature.

Ty and Corey came back to our room for drinks. Tyler and I went for a walk to explore the hotel while the adults chatted like they'd been friends for years. I led the way to the 10th floor balcony that overlooked the beach and ocean.

The view stunned my senses. Ty leaned over the balcony railing and listened to the waves lap along the shoreline. Myrtle Beach, had activities for people of all ages. I gazed out at the moonlit beach and couldn't imagine myself anywhere else.

I wished the date lasted forever. The map teetered into unchartered territory. Once again butterflies danced around my stomach. I reflected on the events of the evening as the light pranced across the waves of the ocean.

A few rowdy kids shouted from the lazy river on the ground floor far below us. The young teenagers somehow got the impression that Ty and I had snuck out for a romantic stroll.

Our connection wasn't anybody's business but our own. I didn't have any idea what the goings on with us meant. Had we just experienced a date? I thought the outing had all the elements of real date. Ty slipped my left hand and into his and continued to walk. In my mind I shrieked with joy. Ty rubbed my fingers. I had to pinch myself.

*****

In 2001, I was a senior in high school. All of my friends chose colleges and universities to attend the following fall.

The key to picking a college or university was discovering what can't live without doing and making that your career. I kept my options open by applying to two universities and three different programs.

Ty determined McMaster best suited his academic career. I plopped my chemistry books down on my desk which happened to be next to him and sighed.

I applied to Brock for two different programs and Guelph for my third choice. Guelph University didn't fit my future plans, but you could apply to three programs, so I chose a school that offered Child and Youth Studies.

I hoped to live in residence at Brock because I didn't drive. I knew the university was close, but I wouldn't do well living far away. I crossed my fingers, that all of my aspirations would come true.

Kelsey Naughton, the oldest of the three children I babysat was aware of the goings on in her household. She usually talked a mile a minute, but something caused her to be down in the dumps. She overheard her parents discussing the possibility of me living in residence.

Kelsey and her brother Theo and sister Natasha, didn't care to have a new babysitter. I had nothing but love for the Naughton kids. Kelsey revealed to me that Theo only combed his hair when I came over.

*****

The summer after high school went by all too fast. In September of 2001, I headed to Brock to get a psychology degree and live in residence.

Bones,

I know you'll do well at Brock. They're fortunate to have you. I'll miss you, but we'll connect when we're home for the holidays.

Have fun Bones. Keep that cute smile on your face. You just smiled. I wish I could see you smiling, but just knowing that you are makes me happy.

Happy move in day to you.

Love,

Ty xo

Oh the mystery of is Tyler. Maybe taking psychology would bring me some understanding of Ty.

*****

In late October of my freshman year, I settled at university. The slight fall breeze, made a perfect setting for walking to class through the outdoor courtyard.

I unraveled what Tyler and I meant to one another. Thanksgiving approached and I still had no clue. I had a great friend now, but I deserved to know if something more could be under the surface.

I had to talk to Tyler and get some answers. The last couple of times we'd been together, I felt like he wanted to tell me important news.

*****

During Christmas break, I was determined to sort through my friendship with Tyler. For my own sanity, I had to discover what our relationship was. Even if we never became a couple, I had to know if I barked up the wrong tree.

Tyler came over to watch a movie and hopefully we'd be able to talk. I peered out the sheer covered bay window of my family's home.

Ty had muscles. I squeezed his rock hard bicep. He was an athletic guy. I couldn't stop smiling. I leaned in to take his coat and caught the scent of his cologne. He smelled incredible. Ty grinned back at me. He said he'd have to borrow my jeans. Tyler spoke to my parents briefly as we passed the living room.

What bothered Tyler? I grabbed two sodas from the bar fridge. Ty played with his fingers.

I thought his bulletin was about his parents. I sat beside him, with only half a couch cushion between us. What he had to say was more about him.

Nicole came by and I introduced Tyler to my sister-in-law. She borrowed my grey pea coat. Chad and Nicole went out to dinner. I told Nicole my jacket should be in the hall closet on the right hand side. Nicole confessed she'd used my deodorant because aroma smelled incredible. I found Nicole hard to read sometimes. I figured the sharing of clothing and deodorant meant we had become true sisters. What's mine was hers and vice versa.

Our family dog hopped up on the half cushion that separated us and lay down. Lassie made herself at home. I snuggled her golden fur. Lassie put her head beside Ty and hunkered down. Lassie set herself between us, as if to let us know I was her girl.

Ty patted Lassie and the dog didn't make a move. What a good boy. Lassie preferred to be part of the action. I placed my hand on her velvet like ear.

I encouraged Ty to speak to me. I held Tyler's free hand and squeezed his shaky digits. Whatever he had to say, we'd figure out together. He scared me.

He goal wasn't to frighten me, but I might not like the words he spoke. He didn't want to lose me. A light bulb turned on inside my head and I knew what he was attempting to tell me.

Ty finally got his words out. He told me that he was gay. Ty had taken a giant leap out of the closet. He whimpered and I hugged him with the dog in between us. Ty struggled to be verbal.

Oh my sweet Tyler. Tears streamed down each of our faces as we sat silently in an intricate ball of emotion. He frantically pet the dog. I tried to understand the ramifications of his words.

Ty almost let me in on his secret several times and backed out at the last minute. I could tell something was on his mind, but I didn't know what. I figured in time Ty would open up and release his secret. I hoped I didn't say the wrong thing in a conversation to him.

The dog lay motionless except for the rise and fall of her back as he breathed. Ty put a handful of dog fur on the end table. Lassie was shedding, if Ty hadn't collected the excess dog hair, clumps of fur would be scattered all over the floor.

He asked if I'd lend him the jeans I was wearing sometime. That comment was a little too soon, but we both laughed. Baby steps would be appreciated. I just found out he's gay. He wouldn't be the groom at my wedding. I tried to frown, but soon returned to smiling. How could I not smile when I peeked at his cute face?

Ty was sorry that he wouldn't be what I wanted him to be. He'd thought about me a lot over the last few months. Ty envisioned us being a couple too, but he had too much affection for me to put me through that when he questioned his sexuality.

Tyler didn't choose to be gay, he just was. He desired the same things I did. Ty dreamed of a partner, a career, a home, kids, and a white picket fence.

Tyler being gay didn't change his physical or mental person. In my eyes, Ty was the same boy he had always been. Sure, he wouldn't be sitting at the head table at my wedding, but I'd move forward. He was going to be a part of my life no matter what.

"People have said I love you are the three hardest words to say. Those people have never had to say I am gay." Ty gently captured my hands in his.

Ty would make a wonderful father one day. From an early age, I'd pictured him handing out orange slices at our kid's soccer game. I thought I would have his children. I had faith in him as a human being.

Ty smiled, lost in his own thoughts. His emotions were raw.

I saw versions of Ty and me running around the soccer field. We'd work things out as they came up, but I jumped way ahead of myself. I broke free from my fantasy dream.

My family thought Ty was wonderful and him being gay wasn't going to alter their opinions of him. I wiped a tear from my cheek. Will and Chad would be fine with Ty being gay. My brothers liked Ty because he was good to me and that's what mattered. My family wasn't going to judge Ty for circumstances beyond his control.

Tyler was himself and that's who he was supposed to be. I would always care for him and he would have a place in my heart. I beamed at him through tears. I had to move him from possible husband to friend. I'd learn how to do that so I didn't lose my Ty forever.

I was unsure when Ty knew he was gay. I stopped crying momentarily. Tyler hadn't known forever. He had his suspicions in high school, but in university he explored his sexuality. Ty went out with a few girls and had zero connection. He made out with one girl to test the waters and the feelings didn't occur. The girl could tell the kiss was not right. Ty let a single tear drop onto the dog.

Thank heaven he didn't choose to explore his sexuality with me. Kissing me wouldn't have ended well. I would wonder if I turned him gay. I peered at Ty through blurred vision.

Ty could never do that to me. He knew if he did kiss me, he might lose me as a friend. Selfishly, Ty had to have me in his life. I realized now I could never turn him gay, but girls would speculate. I batted wet lashes.

I questioned whether his parents and brother knew? I was right when I thought he had to talk about his parents. Ty tried to read my face. He told his Mom. He added his parents lived apart.

"I'm sorry that your parents aren't together. That is hard for a child to deal with at any age. How did your mother react when you talked to her?"

Ty's mother stared at him with her mouth hung open. Once they started chatting and Tyler answered her questions, she was alright. They hugged and cried for so long. Connie was shocked. Ty felt he was in a good place with his Mom now that the surprise had worn off.

Tyler hadn't told his brother. He had to figure out how to tell him. Ty's Dad didn't suspect his son had undisclosed private information. His Mom's lips would be sealed until everybody in the family was aware of Ty's news flash.

I cried again. Shocker. Ty wiped my tears away with his index finger. I would be alright. Sometimes I just had to shed a few tears.

Now we could watch girly movies and cuddle on the couch. That wouldn't screw my mind up at all. I knew when Ty willingly watched decorating shows, he was too good to be true.

We could still do dinner and movies. We could go shopping together. Ty had to shop for a new pair of jeans and thought I would tell him if his butt looked big. Come on. As if staring at his fine ass all day wouldn't be a turn on. He might be gay, but my attraction wouldn't disappear overnight. Tyler's butt was just the right size. Trust me, I'd checked his buns out many a time.

Ty's watch said the midnight hour was upon us. I hoped he'd stay a bit longer. Ty motioned for me to come around the dog and sit on his lap. I was okay. I lifted my head from his shoulder. He smelled so good. I wanted him right despite the fact he wasn't attracted to females.

Ty slowly stood up, tiptoeing so as not to disturb the now snoring dog. We walked to the front hall.

Apparently I made Ty comfortable enough for him to speak from his heart. He let his dimples show and hugged me once more. I reached into the closet and pulled out Ty's coat and breathed in his heavenly mix of cologne and deodorant. Ty's jacket hugged every curve of his torso.

I had Ty's phone numbers and email address, so he told me I shouldn't hesitate to contact him with any questions I thought of after he left. Ty kissed my cheek and turned to leave. He urged me to never forget he loved me.

I loved him too, but I remained speechless. I smiled behind my tear stained face and reddened eyes. I watched through the glass door, while Ty started his car. The winter air surrounded me as he drove off toward home. Tyler was gone.

I shut the front door, leaned back against the steel frame and slid down to the floor. I sobbed for a few minutes before getting up. I ruffled Lassie's fur on my way past the living room chair.

I headed upstairs to bed, making an effort not to sniffle too loud. My Dad opened his bedroom door.

Ty told me that he was gay. I thought his parents separated. Boy was I wrong. I grabbed my Dad and cried into his pyjamas. All my Mother could do was put her arms around me, sitting on the edge of the bed.

I found Ty irresistible, but was sad the romantic possibilities ended. Another good guy lost to the other team. I cried and giggled all at once.

My feelings felt off kilter. My parents both held Ty on a pedestal for being himself and looking after me. Their thoughts on Ty hadn't changed because he was gay. I was glad he told me, but I couldn't seem to stop blubbering.

After Nicole met Tyler, she asked if he was gay. I guess I saw what I wanted to see. She didn't know him and viewed him with fresh eyes.

I figured I should get some rest. I yawned, my mouth hanging open.

I let the steam of a hot washcloth hit my face, I felt a tad better. I should write to Ty once I got ready for bed.

Dear Tyler,

Tonight was a night I'll never forget. I did not expect you to tell me you were gay. The thought had never crossed my mind. At the last second, I figured out what you were trying to convey to me.

My dear Lassie was just what we required tonight. How did she know we would be comforted by her presence? She was older than her years. That gal made tonight easier for both of us.

You said all the right things to me at the right time. I know it wasn't a fun conversation for you to start given our long history. I'm sorry you worried about my reaction to your statement.

I've never known a gay person before, so I'd never had to face my feelings about gay people. I was face to face with my thoughts and gay people are the same as everybody else. Trust me when I say that there was never any doubt in my mind about you. When you told me you were gay, I wanted to hold you and never let go.

I had to put my thoughts on paper, so to speak. I meant every word I said tonight. I loved you yesterday. I love you today. I will love you tomorrow and every day after that.

My parents awakened when you left. They heard me sob and sniffle on my way up to bed. They responded just as I knew they would, with open arms. My Mom and Dad send their hugs.

Love always and forever,

Megan xo

Residence Life

Now that I'm so close to graduating, I reminisced about what it was like when I started university. I took a while to realize my school days had nearly come to a close. By October 16th of 2010, I didn't know what the future held for me. I shouldn't daydream too far ahead. I could easily get my mind stuck wondering what would happen in five years. I couldn't be sure what would occur months down the road, but I guessed all of the new graduates were in the same boat.

The 2001-2002 school years amazed me. I spent my first year living in residence. I learned so much about myself during the first few months. I was taught book learning didn't account for all of education; being social played a major role as well.

While I jetted around campus, I came across all manners of dress. Pyjama pants seemed suitable to wear to class or anywhere else on school grounds for that matter. Slippers counted as shoes when rushing to class. Nobody dared to dress in any clothing, but preppy attire at my secondary school. I reminded myself I wasn't in high school anymore. I contemplated these thoughts while I waited to get my degree.

*****

In July of 2001 I finished high school and was working part-time for the summer at an information booth in the tourist district of Niagara Falls. In my spare time I got ready for university.

Despite living close to a university town, I craved the experience of living on campus, while still being close enough I could go home at the last minute. I had taken a leap of faith and stayed in residence.

Life on campus made me a better person. I believe beyond a shadow of doubt, I am who I am due in part to my year in residence.

*****

At some point in my senior year of high school we had to decide which post secondary institutions we applied to.

Jonah's girlfriend Fiona was a year older than me and had lived in a townhouse style residence at Brock University and she was in high spirits when she talked about her accommodations. I thought I preferred a similar dorm.

My friends went to other colleges and universities for the most part. I secretly hoped Jonah went to Brock and lived in residence. I saw us having afternoon naps together and pigging out on junk food and cotton candy ice-cream from the cafeteria.

I fantasized we would flirt during our psychology lectures. I saw Jonah as a good friend and not potential boyfriend, so our relationship was easy and uncomplicated. He joked that he'd been hit on by teenage girls, single mothers, aunts and older males. Jonah saw the different types of people he attracted, as a badge of honor.

In the end, I probably was better off staying in residence by myself and taking chances on a roommate the school chose. I could make friendships on my own, but never be truly alone because one of my neighbours would be around.

If Jonah had lived on my floor, we would have had an open door policy. If he went to Brock with me, my status would have skyrocketed. Co-ed naps would have been pure bliss.

*****

I wondered what my roommate would be like. Would she be fat, skinny, a diva, a loner, a stoner, gothic, outgoing, or an introvert? I hoped we would have stuff in common.

In my residence, each student had their own room and two people shared a connecting bathroom. Even if I ended up with a dud of a roommate, we only shared a bathroom.

I was leaving home for the first time. Going away to university was the first major step since I started kindergarten. I felt scared, but knew I'd be better for taking risks.

As July turned into August, my time was spent packing for my move to residence. My Mom organized different piles in the living room. She jotted lists of what I had yet to purchase. I normally kept my bedroom neat and tidy, but I walked through the house in a stunned manner.

I started packing some clothes. My Mom said I could leave most stuff on hangers and put a garbage bag over the clothing. I gathered some bags marked for residence and placed the totes in the correct area.

I've never moved before, so I didn't know what to do. My mind scattered information all over my head. Platty, my favourite stuffed animal, a platypus, sat in the undecided pile. I raised one eyebrow and moved Platty into the pile of boxes and luggage to go to residence. My Mom smiled to herself, but knew better than to start an argument when I was stressed.

Yum. My Mom bought me a multipack of lunch type snacks and a selection of small bags of chips. Even if I gained the Freshman Fifteen, I'd still be thin.

Liv came into my room and surveyed the bags and heaps of clothing to pack up. All I had left to do was fold some shirts and put garbage bags over the last few hangers. Olivia settled onto a corner of my bed and began to fold my loose shirts. She was the most organized person I had ever met.

My life changed. I rubbed my stomach, to calm the brewing uneasiness. We finished folding all of my shirts and everything was ready to load into the van in the morning.

Liv had the day off from lifeguarding on my move-in day, so she'd gladly bring a car load to my residence. I figured we would get all of the important items into the minivan. I'd email Olivia once I had moved in. I'd see her at the vendor fair in a few days. I hugged my best friend goodbye, even though she was going to the same school. She commuted in her new car.

Truth be told, we would have been helpful to have Olivia take a carload of bags to residence. In order to make the most of my residence experience, I had to start off without my best friend. I stood in the doorway for a moment, my stomach rumbling out loud. I was nervous and excited all at once.

My room appeared so different. My shelves bare and my closet had an old sweater and a dress still in the dry cleaning wrap. I was used to having my television and computer to entertain me while I fell asleep.

*****

I awoke to September and my whole body was full of anticipation. The countdown was complete. My Dad packed up the minivan with most of my belongings.

The drive took us about twenty-five minutes to get to Brock University and we encountered heavy traffic. I was close to my parents and I got the

Suck It Up Sunshine

residence experience.

My parents and I joined the long line of other families eager to move their kids into residence. "Look at all of the other people," I muttered. One of them was my roommate. The moving line was going to take forever. I tapped my left foot.

*****

If my parents said the word, I'd ditch the line and forget about residence. I became six years old. We moved forward. Slowly, but surely, I'd get to the front of the line. I was afraid I made the wrong decision to live in residence. I wanted my Mom. I leaned my head on my Mother's shoulder.

"That girl just butted in line. Can you believe that?" I commented. My Dad breathed heavily thinking he would relax. I prayed my father wouldn't open his mouth. She could have been my roommate and I wasn't going to start off on the wrong foot. I wiped my sweaty brow with the back of my right hand.

My Mom referred to the girl who skipped part of the line as "Buttinski". My mother injected her humour and made us all giggle.

My father was pleased the line moved. My turn to get my room key had finally arrived. No more waiting for this girl.

My brother Chad and his wife Nicole Scala gave me a phone card which allowed me to call them in Toronto whenever I wanted. I could call home even though I didn't get the long distance phone plan. I'd connect with my friends from high school online through social media.

My Dad pulled up to the unloading zone. We began to load up what we could onto the moving dolly. My father pulled out a laundry basket full of all kinds of my laundry supplies and placed a bunch of boxes on the moving cart the residence provided.

I got a big room, so I was able to use my exercise ball. I bounced on the bed, letting my long legs dangle over the edge. I couldn't believe I had my own bed, desk and so much space in my residence room.

My Mom coaxed me to load my toiletries into the cupboard in the bathroom. My Mom thought her chestnut brown hair might turn gray by the end of the day, as she prodded me to complete a small task.

I hopped up and headed to the bathroom, grabbing a drugstore bag. "Why on earth would I use dental floss?" I grumbled to nobody in particular.

A man leaned into the bathroom from the other residence room. Dr.

Patrick Baxter, a dentist and coincidently my roommate's father. I stood silent, as embarrassment registered on my face. He could tell me lots of reasons why flossing was good for your oral wellness. In the end I used some of the floss to tie a dry erase marker to the white board on my unit door. Sorry.

My mother, Rose, introduced herself. I met my roommate, Morgan Baxter. I had worried about my roommate for most of the summer and now I was standing next to her. I shook hands with Morgan's mother Colleen and her older sister Amber. They had driven in from Kitchener.

The toilet paper supplied by the residence life staff resembled half ply and sand paper was smoother. My Mom brought a few rolls of three ply toilet paper just in case. Toilet paper became number one on the list of items I would soon run out of.

What a day.

The Don for my floor is named Kevin Pellegrino, knocked on my door to tell me our first floor meeting was in thirty minutes in the lounge at the far end of the hall. His dimples showed as he talked. I was already having a blast. The door eased closed as I gave my parents two thumbs up.

The rooms appeared a lot different from when my Dad went to university. His dorm was brand new too. The rooms had been smaller and shared by two people. Bunk beds and two small desks filled each room. The showers and toilets down the hall, and they resembled public pool change rooms. My Mom was happy we didn't open my residence door only to find old and beat up furniture. She would have had trouble leaving me in a mess.

My parents had to admit their little princess was growing up. We had a group hug before I had to leave to go meet the rest of the people I'd be neighbours with for the school year.

*****

Morgan and I walked to the lounge for our hall meeting.

In a newly constructed residence, the lounge furnishings came later, so we made a large oval on the carpet. At least our rooms had furniture. Our Don welcomed the fresh faces to the first ever gathering of the Secord Hall Barracudas.

I thought I saw my roommate across the room, but we'd gone to opposite sides of the room, so I couldn't be sure. Everyone looks like five year olds. We could all use a juice box and a nap. Some animal crackers might be a tasty snack to hold us over until dinner.

My Don was from a suburb of Toronto. We started introducing ourselves one at a time and letting everyone know where we came from.

Nolan and his roommate Easton grew up in Concord, Ontario. Greg roomed across the way from the attractive guy and he hailed from Uxbridge.

Kristoff Lineham came to Brock all the way from Switzerland. The whole room clapped. Most of us pined for home already, but we held ourselves together. Kristoff flew on an airplane in order to attend school and he showed no signs of longing for home.

Theresa was from Paris, Ontario. I stared across the room at the girl who butted in line earlier in the day; Buttinski lived down the hall from me. Heidi drove in from Ancaster. She let Buttinski butt in front of her. I think the two girls shared a bathroom.

Kevin had some notes to go over before we headed over to the cafeteria. After a brief discussion, Kevin stood up and we all followed him like ducklings behind their leader. The residence meet and greet was supposed to be brief, so we could have dinner afterwards.

The Secord Hall Barracudas had a seat on the floor of the cafeteria. I wondered at some point if we would get to sit in actual chairs. Crossing our legs in a circle on the floor reminded me of kindergarten.

The head of residence life talked about rules to do with the cafeteria and each dormitory. A couple more items to talk about and then we could get some grub.

A naked guy ran in front of the microphone, cheering as he ran out the other side of the cafeteria. I couldn't believe what I was seeing. The girls perked up. How cool.

The barbeques had been turned on outside. I hadn't thought about food all day, but I was starving. Hotdogs tasted best when eaten outdoors. I sat with my new neighbour, Alexis Barlow.

When we finished our hotdogs and began the short trek back to our rooms. I wasn't used to all of the walking, but I managed to stay on my feet.

I unlocked my door and surveyed all of the work my parents had done to get my room setup. They moved the book shelf and chest of drawers to suit me better.

Hi Megan,
We hope you like what we did with the furniture. Your TV is set up and there's plenty of cold drinks in your bar fridge. We'll call you later tonight to

see how you're doing.
Don't forget to floss.
Love,
Mom & Dad xo xo

I wasn't sure how I would handle all of the walking just to go to the cafeteria, but I had faith my body would adjust. Thank goodness for physiotherapy. I'd be one fit girl by the end of the residence year.

My parents would be coming up the following day to hook up my Ethernet. I wasn't sure what that entailed, but I had to have one in order to use the internet.

I could call my parents almost anytime and they'd be smiling on the other end. Sometimes I just had to hear their voices.

*****

I shut my door as Alexis stepped into the hall. I awakened in time to go for breakfast. Hash browns and scrambled eggs topped the menu, so I thought I'd mosey on over to the cafeteria. She joined me.

The cook plopped some egg on my plate. I thanked her and moved ahead with my tray. Alexis loaded up her plate and headed to a nearby table. We were both impressed they had chocolate milk.

At first, when I saw the drink station, I pondered how I would get liquid in a plastic cup and then walk to a table without spilling. I learned to fill my tall cup 2/3 full, that way I wouldn't splash liquid all over.

My parents arrived to set up my internet. My Mom and I let my Dad tackle my computer. My mother stopped at the drugstore and got Morgan and me some extra toilet paper. She put an extra roll in the bathroom and stuck the rest in the back of my closet.

Morgan had her slender fingers on her hip with an extra roll of toilet paper in her other hand. The half ply provided was rough to the touch. She wrinkled her nose to indicate her displeasure with the sheer toilet paper. We had been spoiled with the soft three ply our parents used at our respective homes.

We could use the one ply paper as a backup. Morgan's Mom sent some toilet paper as well, so we had a stockpile. Morgan preferred the stuff my mother had put on the roll.

Thirty minutes later, my Dad had my computer working. ICQ was up and running (the social media of the time). I was amazed at all of the people online. Seth was in Montreal, Alana was in British Columbia, Jonah moved to Kingston, and a bunch of friends lived in Niagara. I squealed with excitement and hugged my Dad.

Hello Friends,
I'm away at school. You can still reach me at my hotmail email address.
My snail mail address is:
Alan Earp Residence
Brock University
500 Glenridge Ave.
St. Catharines, ON
Unit 454
CANADA
L2S 3A1
Megan xo

I checked my email and a lot of notes and well wishes overstuffed my inbox.

Dear Megan, Megannnnn, Brina, MacDaddy, Heather McMac and any other nickname I left out,
Football camp went well, although I'm not as good as most of the other guys.
I met a girl named Heather and I called her 'Heather McMac' and she told me to 'Fuck off'. I realized that not everyone is as tolerant as you & Livy are.
You guys put up with Boyd and me all through high school.
You deserve a medal.
Never Change.
Fletch
Jonah Fletcher

I tended to think that Jonah was good at everything he did. The note made me chuckle to myself.

*****

After lunch, I walked over to the vendor fair to meet Olivia as we'd planned. She had lots of questions for me. Liv was curious about my roommate. She couldn't wait to see my dorm room.

I didn't expect to get free stuff, like the teen packs we used to get from the drugstore. I saw a vegetarian club and across the aisle there was a booth advertising the "meatetarian" society. The meat eaters had a banner that read: 'You don't make friends with salad'. I couldn't argue with the slogan because I wasn't a person who found leafy greens tasty.

Liv was happy to see my new digs. I had a copy of my schedule for my best friend. I expected we would find a time and place to have lunch together.

Mondays at noon would work for both of us to meet for lunch once lectures and seminars began. Olivia compared the typed lists. We agreed to meet in the tower cafeteria.

*****

I craved snack food. I decided to invite Morgan over for some roommate bonding. Morgan stood up from her spot on the floor where she'd been unpacking some books and movies. She grabbed a package of breadsticks that you dip in cheese. We each had a case of similar lunch snacks.

I started to open up to my roommate. Morgan and I learned that we were both the babies of our respective families. Being the smallest child meant that we were both little princesses. How did I manage to get a roommate that was so similar to me? I don't remember filling out a survey that tried to match people based on their likes and dislikes. The university couldn't have given me a better roommate.

My residence experience was shaped by meeting Morgan and clicking from the beginning. We each had other friends and were independent enough that we didn't get tired of one another. Maybe God placed us side by side because He knew we'd be good for one another.

*****

I considered going to the tie-dye activity, but nobody else was available to attend the event. My roommate continued to organize her closet. I had unpacking to do too, but I left the bins for later. Nothing said I couldn't go on my own. I'd take the pillowcase with, "what dreams are made of" printed on the front. The residence life staff gave each student one on move-in day.

In the late morning I made the short walk to the tie-dye social. The head resident showed us how to tie-dye our own items. Once we had dip died our items, we left the pillowcases and t-shirts to dry on a clothes line in a courtyard.

I went back to my room and phoned home. Living in residence turned out to be a superb choice for me. The food plan was exceptional. The buffet of choices was a food dream. Shout out to my parents. They had me settle on simple selections, so I would know what to do when I had several options.

Everyone I dealt with stopped to chat. I had to thank my parents for helping to me get to the point where living in residence was not just a possibility, but a reality.

I decided if I arrived in the cafeteria and didn't see familiar faces, I'd sit with other people and introduce myself. Most of the kids living on campus didn't recognize too many people either.

*****

Hi Megan,
I hope you have a ball at university. My meal plan was yummy. Eat until you're full and don't worry about your weight. Even if you gained the freshman fifteen, you'd still be teeny tiny.
I'm an email away.
Daphne

I caught forty winks before dinner. Morgan was up for a rest too, so we'd have a late supper together. She pulled a blanket over herself and set her book on her night table.

The pasta primavera looked and smelled incredible. I picked up the hot ramekin. Morgan set her tray next to Alexis and her roommate Dana Cederholm.

The bathroom vents go out into our hall. You could tell when you came to a boy's room. They didn't smell as flowery as the girls' rooms. Morgan made a funny face as we walked toward our rooms. Our bathroom had an aroma of lilacs. I sniffed the air.

I unlocked my door and the phone rang. I set my bag down and answered the phone to hear my brother Will. He had talked to our Mom earlier in the day. She started to talk about me and cried a little. My Mother was over the moon I was having a good time in residence. She had uneasiness because I didn't live at home anymore.

"Mom never cries," I note the sadness surrounding my words. Will conveyed just how much she missed me. I sniffled. He didn't mean to make me cry. Mom would be alright.

A moment later there was a knock at my door. I wiped a lone tear from my cheek. The temperature in our rooms seemed a bit warm. Morgan turned the thermostat down. She walked into my room. I proposed we break out some cold drinks. Morgan smiled and pounced onto my bed. The following day a few of the girls explored the campus to find out the locations of the lecture halls classrooms.

*****

Looking at my schedule, Thistle, seemed the place where lectures took place. Room three hundred and twenty five remained a mystery. I glanced up at the other girls in confusion.

Dana flagged a janitor and even he didn't know. We found an elevator to take us to the third floor, but we didn't see any stairs. To be honest, taking the elevator was fine by me. I didn't care if we ever found the stairs.

The ladies filed into the elevator. We tried each button because the number pad had no three listed. When the doors opened, I saw a sign for the classroom, but no staircase. We elected to take the elevator the first day and see where people headed when they filtered out of the class.

*****

Hi Daphne,
I didn't know how much fun living in residence would be. You were right, the meal plan is fantastic.
I'm nervous about the workload, but I guess that is fairly common.
The distance between classes has me slightly concerned, but for that reason my lectures and tutorials aren't ever back to back. I can stop for a donut when I have a break. The Canadian maple is my favourite so far.
My life is full of good cheer.
Megan

Nicole phoned to see how my first day of class went. I walked pretty far to get from class to class. My day went well. I had tortellini with alfredo sauce baked in cheese and some raw veggies and dip for dinner. She was apprehensive I maintain my weight or even gain some. I was so skinny and she worried I'd get enough nutrition. I would be expending a lot more energy than when I went to high school.

Morgan was grateful I'd be home on Monday afternoon. Around two o'clock I'd be available. Her computer was to be delivered by the bookstore and she wouldn't be around to let them in. I didn't mind hanging out in her room to let them in and be available while the bookstore staffer hooked up the internet.

*****

Nobody prepared for what happened on September 11th 2001.

I could hear my phone ringing. Surely I imagined the sound. I didn't have a class on Thursday until mid-afternoon. The noise persisted so I figured the call must be important.

When I picked up the phone, my Mom instructed me to turn on my television. Any channel was fine. The same horrific scenes aired on various channels. What was going on? I could only speculate.

The World Trade Center in New York City had been hit by a plane. Media coverage showed a few citizens staggering out of the building. The news came through unedited and gruesome. The second tower of the World Trade Center was hit by another plane while I sat in silence on the phone.

Morgan woke up confused as to why the same show was playing on every channel we got. We stared at the television in disbelief. People jumped out of windows to try to escape. The media soon reported the planes that hit the towers resulted from a terrorist attack.

The world would never be the same. The news depicted the chaos happening as people ran for their lives.

I struggled to return to my life at school. Sluggish students walked around, stunned looks on their faces. Everywhere you turned, the reporters replayed the moment when the tower went down. The world was at war. My heart filled with sadness.

I returned to my studies to lose myself in my books. Blocking the news out was a survival mechanism.

*****

My mind fluttered with dreadful images. My heart broke for the horrific times ahead for the United States of America.

In the wake of the tragedy, I wrote to do lists for each day, so I didn't forget to do important chores.

My Monday jobs included sheet exchange day. You handed in dirty sheets and received clean ones back. What a deal. I offered to get Morgan some fresh sheets.

Although Liv came and went to my room, she wasn't a permanent fixture in my dorm. A girl in my hall had a friend who drove to class everyday and during breaks she hung out in Dana Cederholms's room. I wondered how this affected her relationship with her roommate, but that was their business.

*****

Friday arrived and Olivia came to spend the night. I made sure Morgan felt welcome to join us, but she had planned to go home that weekend.

Livy phoned to say she was leaving home and would be at my place in about twenty minutes. She had picked me up, so I could lend a hand to carry her bags back to my room. She left her car in the free parking area because the school frowned upon overnight parking in the paid lots.

"Oh no." I paused as I stepped onto the lawn beside the residence with a bag on each arm. Olivia had an odd look on her face. Some well dressed staff had gathered in the fireside lounge on the first floor. The booze bottles clinked every stride I took. I was considered underage. I'd be old enough to drink alcohol in November. We stopped for a minute to reorganize the bags. Olivia had turned nineteen the previous June, so she lifted the cloth bag of vodka mixed drinks and walked forward.

Liv thought we could decorate my room with some pictures from home. I brought a life size poster of Michael Jordan that had been Chad's, to brighten up the cinder block walls. I also got some glow-in-the-dark stars to brighten up my ceiling. Liv and I got set to cover my room in pretty items.

Morgan came back, but without her toothbrush. I had an extra one, but my dentist's name stamped on the side. Morgan promised not to tell her Dad. She went back to the bathroom to brush her teeth.

*****

My schedule on Thursdays allowed me to sleep in and feast on the residence cafeteria macaroni and cheese at lunch. I gathered from the online menus that meals ran on a two week rotation. Every other Thursday the students ate nachos and hotdogs at noon.

111

The food the school sites offered often graced my computer screen. I snacked throughout the day and evenings. Morgan had basically the same eating patterns as me, one of the many reasons we made such great roommates.

"Survivor" was supposed to air after commercials. Morgan and I settled in to watch the first episode of the season. "Seriously?" I yelled in a frustrated tone. A presidential speech interrupted "Survivor". We both grew irritated.

Chad and Nicole came to see me. Nicole thought my room was much bigger than her dorm room. Mom said Chad and Nicole would take my laundry home, so I set a bag by the door. Nicole pointed through the open bathroom door. She had to meet my roommate.

My classes required a lot of reading each week, but generally the topics interested me. Since Boyd wasn't going to school until January, I invited him over after dinner on his day off. Morgan and I liked to watch "Pop Stars" on Thursday evenings. I told Boyd he couldn't date my roommate. Besides, Boyd wasn't her type. I introduced Morgan to my friend Boyd. I mouthed the word "no" to Boyd.

*****

Summer had faded into early autumn. October arrived and I developed a routine with my classes. I learned to wear my backpack with the straps over both of my shoulders and the "seatbelt" done up to ease the stress on my back from carrying my books to and from classes.

I knew I could go home whenever I wanted to. If I decided to stay, my family understood. Sometimes I went home, so I could rest my muscles.

My neighbour Alexis could be a bit clingy. On Mondays I met Olivia for lunch in the tower café. Alexis didn't go to the residence cafeteria for lunch on those days very often. She had become a good friend, but we both had other friendships. Part of university or college is being able to make new relationships in many areas of your life.

I really hoped Morgan still had the sample deodorants from the vendor fair because I left my deodorant at home on the weekend. She did and I could take them all. Morgan saved me from stinking. I'd go over to the campus corner store on my way home from my classes the next day and pick up some deodorant.

Residence Life Part 2

The people on the stage readied themselves for the students to receive their degrees. I spent some of the best moments of my life at Brock University. I'd mark another fabulous life moment. I checked out the gym in all directions, captivated by the pomp and circumstance surrounding the audience.

I slipped back into the year I lived in residence.

*****

I'd officially been at university for a bit over month. I enjoyed my psychology course. I also liked the linguistics course more than I thought I would. My English professor led an eccentric life to say the least. For our independent projects we could bake brownies or do a collage to go along with our essay. I took pleasure in expressing my artistic side. Most of my courses interested me, so homework wasn't a chore.

My Grandma McIntyre sent me a letter. The paper smelled like lavender with a hint of old crayons. As I read her note my eyes began to well up and silent tears fell down my cheeks as I sat on the edge of my bed. My Grandma's brother had been the mayor of St. Catharines and was instrumental in getting Brock University built where it currently stands.

When the university opened, they honoured my Great Uncle Nelson with an honorary degree. My Grandma saved the invitation to the ceremony for many years. She mailed the typed page to me, thinking I might find the invitation meaningful now that I attended Brock.

I kept the letter tucked away in my desk drawer while I was in residence. The message from my Grandma inside a faded envelope meant the world to me. My grandmother was a big fan of post-secondary education. Her children and now grandkids made her one proud Mama. My Grandma had to deal with a thyroid problem after high school; which meant she couldn't continue with her education. When her granddaughters reached high school age, she encouraged us to keep going in whatever field fascinated each one of us.

*****

Brownies were warm and gooey, but brownies soaked in Kahlua were amazing. My Mom made "Death by Chocolate" and sent some back to residence with me. On a Monday morning after our Science lecture, Morgan and I had a sweet treat. If we didn't tell anybody, there'd be more dessert for us. Morgan rubbed her hands together. I knew she'd like the chocolate part because we were keen on most of the same food.

*****

I didn't mind science class, but the early lectures weren't my favourite. I was taking the class in order to satisfy the science course requirement of my program. I was interested in the section we did on pig stem cell transplants in humans with Parkinson's disease. If there was a development in any neuromuscular disease, the results could be of interest to other neurological disorders.

Daphne,
I'm learning lots about myself in my psychology class.
My science professor has been talking about stem cells. Not to worry though,
I'm not on a waiting list to have pig stem cells transplanted into my body. The
subject is interesting.
Megan

Even if the positive discoveries weren't directly linked to Friedreich's Ataxia, the findings may give clues to unlocking other neurological mysteries.

The air smelled of wet soil after a rainfall. Morgan danced down the sidewalk leading to our building. She was awfully cheerful for it still being morning. A snack awaited us back in my room.

*****

I couldn't believe Thanksgiving was near. I continued to pack for my long weekend at home as I chatted with Morgan. My Canadian history lecture was cancelled for that Friday, so I could head home after my science lecture.

I put on my backpack and almost fell backwards due to the weight of my books. My Mom picked up the big bag and we began the short walk to the car. One of my neighbours stopped to give me a big hug and he wished me a Happy Thanksgiving. After our brief hug Sammy was on his way. He was a drama major and quite possibly gay, but we all know that my "gaydar" needs a tune-up. My Mom could wipe away any thoughts of an undisclosed relationship.

I was home. I wasn't sure why my high school graduation was on the Friday evening of the long weekend. At least we wouldn't sweat to death in a gymnasium without air conditioning. I couldn't wait to get the ceremony over with. Balance in a crowd of people wasn't one of my strong suits. My eyes were watery and filled to the brim with emotions.

The master of ceremonies called out my name. I was glad he didn't say Brine. My English teacher, Mrs. Dovers, handed me my diploma. I received my diploma and managed not to fall flat on my ass. A lone tear ran down the side of my face. The guy in front of me had offered to trip, so he'd be known as the person who went down during our graduation ceremony.

Relief spread through my body. I was worry free on a three day weekend. Liv and I had to log some time with our guys while we were all home from university.

I was so happy to see Jonah. I even had makeup on, so the post-graduation photos would shimmer. Boyd was full of energy because his best buds were in Niagara once again.

Once I came back to residence, my Mom put away my clean laundry before she and my Dad left for home. I puttered about putting my books away. Morgan made tea and we got caught up on each other's weekend happenings.

*****

Morgan came to Brock University thinking she was going to become a teacher. She wasn't sure what career she was cut out for. Morgan contemplated packing her stuff and heading home. She didn't realize the university was full of young people who changed their mind about which program they should be in, or which job was the ultimate goal.

Morgan's parents urged her to do some research and find out what other people planned to do with their Child and Youth Studies degree. Morgan thought career services would be helpful. In fact the career services office had binders for each program that listed the jobs people became involved in after their time at Brock.

Breaking in a new roommate wasn't something I contemplated doing. Morgan was fabulous. We were used to each other's schedules. What was I supposed to do now? I wasn't positive anything I could say would make her stay, but I had to at least throw out some ideas.

Morgan fidgeted as she stared at me. My dream was to be a child life specialist; a form of play therapy for children admitted to the hospital, or who were having a procedure done at an outpatient clinic.

I told her in order to be a child life specialist one had to have either a three year degree in child and youth studies or psychology. After a degree was achieved, you required a one year post-grad diploma program at McMaster University that included two work placements.

Morgan sat on the edge of my bed with her elbows on her knees and her chin resting in her hands, listening to me with a slight smile brewing.

When I was fifteen I had surgery on my back. I recalled my pre-op appointment. Prior to surgery I met with a child life specialist. The lady explained what would happen and I had a look at where I would stay after surgery. The lady seemed to be dedicated to her job.

After surgery, there was a child life specialist on duty to talk with patients, play with children and run fun activities geared at specific age groups. I decided while I was in the hospital that I aspired to be a child life specialist.

Morgan and I talked for a long time. She knew after our chat she belonged at Brock University and was indeed in the right program. Phew, that was a close call. Morgan and I had grown into an easy-going friendship. Not all roommates develop into lifelong friends.

*****

I phoned my mother to see how her Hallowe'en prep was going. She was carving a pumpkin without me. We hadn't carved a pumpkin in a few years because we had a foam jack-o-lantern. I sniffled and dabbed my eyes with a tissue because I wasn't at home to assist my mother in carving the pumpkin.

I had to hand out candy to the kids as I'd done in the past. I wasn't old enough to go to any bars or pubs that were hosting Hallowe'en costume parties. My Mom was kind enough to pick me up for the evening. I know it's silly, but the four year old inside me had to be giving out candy on Hallowe'en with my Mommy.

*****

The next day, I tore off the October calendar to reveal November. A neon orange post-it indicated I had received a package larger than my mailbox. I missed the hours the mail room was open to collect my parcel. I had to wait until the following Monday when the residence post office opened up again. What a bummer.

The weekend was filled with wonder as I pondered what could be in the box someone had sent to me. I handed the slip of paper to the older student sitting behind a table in the mailroom. The brown cardboard carton had a return address I hadn't heard of before. Maybe they gave me the wrong container.

Alexis and I sat down on a bench in the residence lobby to open up my mail. I pulled out a plastic lizard and knew creature had a story.

Dear Megan,
We were at Walmart and Zack spotted the lizard and knew we had to mail it to you.
We hope you two get along.
Your favourite neighbours,
Zack & Mia Sweeton
P.S. The return address was Zack's work to confuse you.

Lizzy the lizard was so ugly she was cute. I placed the green and yellow amphibian on the top of the bookshelf next to my boom box. Morgan giggled at the life-like creature.

I took pictures of the lizard in my dorm room. Lizzy the lizard came home with me for a weekend visit. The hunk of plastic was having quite the time at school. Mia's daughter would likely going to McMaster University following year and living in residence. Addie would receive the lizard in the mail. I would add photos and a journal before I mailed Lizzy to Addie.

Lizzy was good company and didn't require any work on my part. She didn't eat me out of house and home, which was great because Morgan and I appreciated our snack food, especially sweets.

*****

My parents couldn't believe their baby girl was turning nineteen on November 11th, 2001. Banana cake with peanut butter icing was a traditional birthday dessert in my family. My Mom made some cupcakes for me to take back to residence. Morgan was interested in a banana cupcake with peanut butter icing. She'd eat anything my Mom baked.

Morgan and I couldn't get warm. She made tea to warm us up. Tea and cake fit for two princesses. I silently wondered if all of the other rooms seemed as cold as ours. Alexis' room always felt hot. I held my mug of tea with gloves on. I didn't do well in extreme heat because my mother kept our house cool year round.

Will picked me up in fifteen minutes to go to the casino. I put some lip balm on my chapped lips and went down to the residence lobby to wait inside because the weather was frosty. Will wasn't permitted to gamble because he was an employee on the gaming floor. Will turned on the heated seats in his car to warm us up.

Inside the casino the temperature was just right. A middle-aged man with red suspenders and navy sweat pants spoke from his chair at a black jack table. He wondered what Will was doing at work on his day off.

I didn't like the carpet in the casino that ran the span of the building. I couldn't flash my eyes in the general direction of the ground. The carpet didn't contain any straight lines for me to follow. I tried to focus on my brother.

The carpet was a busy design, so people wouldn't look down. The bright lights in the ceiling keep you from turning your head toward the sky. Therefore the players kept their eyes on the gaming floor. A customer's eyesight should be level with the slot machine because when somebody wins the casino benefits by having other people take notice.

*****

Morgan knocked on my bathroom door and I lost my balance. Shit. I stubbed my toe on the door stop. A fall was bound to happen with the doorstop being in the middle of the room. I sat down on my desk chair.

Morgan spotted the Ziploc bag she wanted. We never shut the bathroom doors except when we used the washroom. We shared items back and forth all the time. I had only met Morgan at the start of the year, but we had a mutual trust.

Morgan and I walked back to residence after dinner one night. A girl in a power wheelchair stopped us in our tracks.

The girl was curious to know if I had the wheelchair room on the fourth floor. She didn't give her name or say hello. How rude of her to speak to us like she owned the joint. She demanded to know where I grew up. I refrained from telling her it was none of her fucking business.

I refused to call her a lady because she wasn't one. In her opinion, people from Niagara Falls shouldn't be allowed to live in residence because the city was too close to the university.

Her friend from Sault Saint Marie didn't get into residence. If I wasn't supposed to live on campus, the university wouldn't have accepted my application. Getting a dorm room was a lottery system and I got my room fair and square. I gave a fake half smile at the nameless girl and kept on walking.

I couldn't believe that girl. What right did she have to question me about where my family resided? Morgan suggested we refer to her as Scootie.

I had some wine coolers left over from when Olivia stayed over. Morgan put her dark curly hair into a loose ponytail as she peered in my fridge to see what flavours of alcohol I had left. We each cracked a bottle open. The school week was over and we had to decompress after our run in with Scootie. Meet the Fockers seemed to be on a continuous loop on HBO. The movie credits just started, so we grabbed some pillows and got comfortable. We clinked glasses and had a prolonged sip of our drinks.

On our way to brunch the next morning Alexis and I chatted. She could hear me and Morgan laughing last night. I was not impressed with her inquisition. We didn't yell or do anything disruptive. We had a drink or two while we viewed television and talked. Morgan and I were generally quiet people. We didn't blast our music or scream and swear in our rooms. The person above had plenty of sex with the bed too close to the wall, but the noise wasn't worthy of a complaint.

Alexis had a sensitive personality, so Morgan and I had to tread lightly. Neither one of us set out to specifically leave Alexis out. We couldn't change how she dealt with certain situations, so we had to move on from this incident. Besides, we had become friends with Alexis.

The end of our fall semester was less than a week away. Morgan pulled up the December exam schedule on my computer. Of course my classes crammed in at the end of the timetable. Perhaps a good night's sleep would make my midterm arrangement appear to be better than my reality.

*****

A knock at the door came one morning. I wore my plaid flannel pyjamas and a sweatshirt over top because I froze otherwise. My Don informed me the final inspection of our rooms would be the next morning. Kevin examined the notes scribbled on his yellow legal pad. Our schedules permitted me to be home during the visit from the project managers.

The lady inspector thought our bathroom fan sounded like a lawn mower. She wrote something on her clipboard paper. I nodded my head. The fan just started sounding loud few weeks ago

The temperature in our rooms was cold no matter what we set the thermostat at. In the beginning of the school year our rooms left us constantly warm, but since winter began we hadn't been able to keep warm. Morgan and I assumed all of the residences maintained a hot temperature in the summer and colder in the winter months.

The lady said our heating and air conditioning didn't work the way the climate control system should. The repairman would be in to fix the problems later that afternoon.

Why didn't we ask about the cold? We hadn't lived in residence before. But even if we had, our residence was brand new and we had no comparisons.

*****

All I had to do was hit print and I would be done my last essay of the fall semester. Shit. The ink ran out. I prayed Morgan knew how to change the ink cartridge on my printer. I had a new cartridge, but I didn't have a clue on how to change it. My Dad always did the switch when I ran out of ink at home. Maybe instead of being a princess, I should have paid attention to the moving.

Morgan was a lifesaver. What would I do without her?

Classes had ended for the semester and everyone either studied or wrote essays. Some people finished writing exams before I had even began. Outside my residence room I could see my friends pack up their cars and leave for the holidays.

Morgan and I both had the science exam for non-science people on the last day. We observed other students pack up their clothes and wished everyone a Merry Christmas.

Olivia learned the hard way you should sit at the front of the gym during an exam. Otherwise, every time someone in front stands up, you'll look up and lose your concentration.

Before any exam began each student had to fill out an identification card and place the thick paper the top right hand corner of the desk.

I drew a blank. What did given name mean? A motherly woman nearby eased my worries. A given name was the name your parents gave you.

Well, I made it through my first set of university exams. My Dad loaded my last bag into the van. My family was glad I had a wonderful experience with residence during the first half of the school year.

*****

A new year had begun. January of 2002 was nearly two thirds over. I got a VCR for Christmas. Not everyone remembered life before the DVD and Blu-Ray technologies. My big room was perfect to have people over for a movie night. Morgan had a selection of movies. I had never seen Love and Basketball. I hit play and hopped up on my bed with the other girls.

The next morning on the way to brunch, Alexis began a new discussion. She was shocked at the number of mini chocolate bar wrappers on my bed when someone flicked on the lights once the movie had completed.

Morgan and I ate most of them. I offered the candy to everyone else, but only a few people had one or two. Whatever Morgan and I ate didn't seem to add weight to our petite frames.

Morgan and I were skinny-mini snack people. I wasn't sure how many calories consumed on any given day. I'd lost weight because of the anxiety I had over my exams. I knew one day I would watch what I ate, but I didn't have to count every morsel.

*****

I heard voices coming from Morgan's room. I listened and felt confident the lady speaking was her Mother. She wouldn't be at our dorm in the middle of the week. I decided to get ready for science class.

Morgan knocked on the bathroom door. She had to skip science that morning. She suffered with stomach pain, so her Mom came in the night to take her to the hospital. She could borrow my notes after class. I suggested she pick out any snacks I had. Ginger ale made my tummy less queasy and I had a stock in my fridge.

My Mom felt bad Colleen drove all that way in the night to take Morgan to the hospital. I passed on the message to Morgan that my Mom would gladly take her to the doctor or the hospital. The time of day or night didn't matter. My family was closer to the university than her parents.

I rubbed my eyes and saw my alarm clock said six in the morning. Morgan held her middle and I knew she hurt. She was just shy of being desperate and she needed medical attention. I phoned my Mom and she readied herself to go in no time at all.

I put on some warm-up pants and my 'Barracuda' sweatshirt and I set to leave. Morgan thanked my mother for coming. She managed only a few words while getting into the van. If I lived in Kitchener, Morgan's parents would do the same for me.

Morgan saw the doctor at the hospital. She had a prescription to drop off. Surely a drugstore opened early nearby. The hours posted in the drug store window said the doors would be unlocked at eight. Morgan slid back in the van. We could get a hot drink while we waited for the store lights to come on.

Morgan indicated we didn't have to stay until eight. She bent down and let out a soft moan. My Mom and I couldn't leave her in an unfamiliar plaza by herself. My Mom turned around to face Morgan and gave her a slight smile. Morgan appreciated the company.

The doctors felt Morgan had a stomach bug of some sort. Once she started taking the antibiotics they prescribed, she'd stop having severe bouts of stomach cramps.

*****

February was a drab month. Brock University had little snow piles at the edge of the sidewalks.

Will worked nights at the casino. After his shift one day he met me for breakfast at eight. Will hadn't eaten in a while, so he was happy breakfast was "all you could eat". He grabbed a muffin and three strips of bacon. In the end Will had some eggs and hash browns to round out his plate.

Will grinned. He was proud of me for accomplishing all I had done. I took a risk by moving to residence. Clearly, living on campus agreed with me. Having breakfast with my older brother got my day underway bright and early.

Will wondered about the odd duck in the back corner: he motioned toward the guy eating alone. He and his brother both lived in residence, so

I wasn't sure which one he was. His name was either Garth or Darth. What kind of parent does that to a kid? He had a loon on his sweatshirt, which was bad enough. Rhyming names didn't seem cool for emerging adults. Their mother was a family doctor for crying out loud. She gave medical advice to her patients. One might think she should have some idea of how a person's name can affect their life.

Will's jaw dropped. The guy in the corner put on an "Elmer Fudd" hunting cap and did up the straps under his chin. Will's eyes opened wide in astonishment. He made me laugh whenever we were together.

The braided ponytail who sat in the corner of the cafeteria seemed too old for residence. He might have been part of the construction team. Now the whole table thought I had a not so secret attraction to this unknown male.

He was old enough to be my father. He had a braided rat tail. The loose hair formed of a mullet combo. Since nobody knew his name, we made the decision to call him Brady. Brady Ratullet, to be exact.

*****

I spent the days from Labour Day to Christmas break moving my belongings in. After the holidays I tidied my room and gradually moved my stuff home.

The spring exam schedule released online and I crossed my fingers for a spaced out timetable. I wrote science for non-science people on the last day. Shit.

Time sped by and before long March was upon us. The ice and snow had all but disappeared and the temperature rose with each passing day. Morgan and I finally learned to use our air conditioning and we felt blissfully cool.

My freshman year neared the end. I'd met great people along the way. I tried to remain upright, so I forgot about dating. Attractive guys roomed all the floors of my residence. I didn't want to explain my medical history on a first date.

Nolan was my type I thought. The athletic guy across the hall had my undivided attention. I had become better friends with him. His roommate had a six pack. I could've... would've... should've...

A study room located at the center of my floor had a lot of use during the exam schedule. A group of girls from my floor decided to hold a psychology study group. Dana posted a sign on our hall bulletin board.

*****

Our rooms had to be inspected before we moved out. I hoped my room passed muster. I dropped my mascara wand on the carpet, but I scrubbed the stain out of the rug.

Boyd returned from school. He was eager to make my move home easier. I could use a tall person to take down my glow in the dark stars. While he visited me maybe he could take some pictures of my friends and me. Boyd called me Megannnnnnn and I became homesick.

Boyd wasn't surprised I still had a wide selection of snacks. I was the Snack Master. Studying makes you hungry, so I had lots of possibilities. I went to the campus store and bought some Dr. Pepper, just for Boyd. I liked the cherry flavoured cola too.

A knock at the door and Boyd opened the door a crack. "Megan and I are high school sweethearts. Megan's a little tied up right now because we're getting reacquainted."

I couldn't see who was at the door. I didn't have friends with benefits. Nor were we getting back into our groove sexually the way he'd implied. Suddenly I didn't miss his attitude.

Monica Bien stood in front of my door and appeared to be utterly confused. She had come over to get some pictures with the girls in my hall. Monica had never met Boyd because she lived in another residence building. Morgan was familiar with Boyd's antics and handed him her camera.

I came out to the hall in a minute. "Boyd isn't my boyfriend. He is a friend from high school who has a twisted sense of humor." I stared at Boyd, goose bumps had formed up and down my pale arms.

Boyd hollered at us to say the word sex and snapped photos on a bunch of different cameras. Surprise. Boyd was goofy, but somehow adorable.

Everyone in my residence hall threw in ten dollars at the beginning of the year, so we could have a television in the lounge. Our Don put all the contributor's names in a hat and chose a name.

Kenora Joe informed my lunch table Fat Faith won the television. Big Faith? Silence fell among the girls. We only had one Faith on our floor.

"Relax, I meant fat with a ph because she's a cool chick." Joe informed the now smiling group of ladies. I expected my nickname to be Skinny Meganie.

*****

Classes wrapped up at the start of April. My friends trickled home from school and I hadn't written an exam yet. I just had to get through the five days exams were packed into.

I answered my phone and heard Olivia chatting about coming to see me. Jonah brought Xander Rods and Austin Kelvin home from school with him, so they'd be among the visitors. They wouldn't stay long because I had an exam the next afternoon. My body anticipated a massive hug and I became nervous.

Jonah entered and in his rugged way voiced my nickname. I had missed anyone calling me MacDaddy when talking to me. Jonah lifted me off my feet while I squealed inwardly.

Shit. I was over the moon to see Jonah. I yearned to be in his company. Whether he had a girlfriend or not, his natural sociability and handsome physique made you do a double take.

A large box of Popsicle sticks tucked in on my bottom shelf of my bookcase. I made tea and stirred in the powdered creamer. I didn't want to get into the other uses for the stirrers.

The tongue depressors also helped to mix my creatine powder into a drink. My body doesn't process iron well and as a result, I had excess iron lying around. Creatine was an iron keylator, meaning the powder wraps around the clumps of iron and disposes of it properly. I didn't come up with this cocktail on my own; Dr. Sutton prescribed creatine and a series of vitamins and antioxidants. The bottle of creatine hid under my bed, so nobody would go on a quest for answers.

Jonah made a couple of arrows, one for me and he kept one for himself. Liv emailed me later to tell me that Jonah had put the arrows in the light within the elevator of my building. Jonah left a reminder he had been there. Now every time the elevator arrived, I grinned.

I made mental notes of the items that were mine (like the bulletin board) and what was school property. My Dad used Velcro to hold the framed piece of cork to the cement wall. My Mom's craft paint would hide any markings left behind.

Morgan came into my room to thank my mother for being her Mom away from home. Morgan handed her a box of chocolates. Dr. Baxter appeared grateful that my Mom looked out for his daughter. My Mom had a mothering instinct.

My Mom wished I'd stand next to the residence sign and she'd take my picture. At the time I felt like it was a lame idea. My Mom thought ten years from that moment, I'd be glad I had the picture. I happened to be wearing my Barracudas sweatshirt. My mother got her camera out and adjusted the zoom before snapping the photo.

I had to move forward in life, but for a moment I stayed still. The wind caught my hair and made for a Hollywood style photo. I couldn't believe my year in residence was over. Time flew by in the blink of an eye.

*****

From the front row of my convocation I beamed a toothy smile as thoughts of my freshmen year flowed through my mind. I was full of anticipation.

My Nieces & Nephew

I expected to be finished the ceremony by now and eating a celebratory dinner with my family. I celebrated my special day.

*****

In December of 2003 my family was getting ready for Christmas. The carols played as we decorated for the holidays.

Chad readied himself to ask Nicole to marry him. He talked to her Dad and received approval from her parents.

Chad had his Michael Jordan engagement boxers on. He set out to propose to Nicole. Chad had practiced getting down on one knee in front of tables and chairs in our house. Now he had to do the real deal.

Nicole said yes. I was getting a new sister-in-law. I would finally have the sister I'd always wanted.

Nicole and Chad knew what they had in mind for their wedding. The two set to work on planning the event. They had a short engagement. May 25th, 2004 was the special day.

Chad and Nicole exchanged their vows outdoors at a picturesque winery in Niagara-on-the-Lake, in front of sixty family members and close friends.

*****

Chad and Nicole got a puppy. I was an Auntie to a puppy. Chad hollered and everyone came running to the living room to meet Riley, an English golden retriever. How could anyone look at a pup and not smile? Nicole still had the glow of a newlywed, holding the squirmy little guy in her arms. Riley's fur turned a white blonde colour.

Chad and Nicole received their puppy in the spring, so they could train him over the summer before the snow came and made life difficult. Nicole had heard having a puppy was great training for having children. Riley had a lot of people to give him the attention he craved.

I'd rub Riley's belly for hours so I could see his right leg twitch. What a perfect addition to our family. I believe your happiness should never be in someone else's hands. However, a puppy does increase my positive energy.

In August Riley graduated from his second round of puppy school. Chad and Nicole referred to themselves as Mommy and Daddy. My nephew uplifted everyone's spirits. Chad and Nicole lived in Toronto, but they came over most weekends. Having a puppy in the house brought out the silly side of my family.

My parents didn't mind if Riley had a dip in the pool. As long as he used the steps in the shallow end to get in, I didn't see why Riley couldn't swim. He had a buzz cut, so his fur wouldn't be an issue for the skimmer.

I adored watching my boy swim. I was supposed to start an online course on the first of the month. I didn't have a class to attend, so I could enjoy the summer weather I had material to work on at my own pace. I stretched out on a lounge chair in the semi-shade in front of our pool and squinted toward Riley.

*****

Christmas had come and gone all too fast. Santa brought Riley a package of orange hockey balls to run after in the pool the following summer. I wondered what the year 2005 would bring. I was twenty-two years old and spring was on the way.

In the beginning of May, Chad announced he and Nicole were coming over the next weekend. Chad and Nicole often came over for the day, so nobody suspected ulterior motives.

Chad and Nicole had six months until parenthood. The secret had almost slipped out more than once, but they kept the news to themselves for three months. Soon a baby would be joining our family. I adored being an Auntie to Riley. Happy tears filled my eyes.

My mother was curious to know whether the baby would be a boy or a girl. Chad had to find out. He knew that the ultrasound technician would know the gender of their baby, whether they chose to find out or not.

My Mom made a baby quilt for the baby. It would be helpful to her, if she knew the baby's gender. Nicole and Chad would let everyone know the baby's gender and his or her middle name. No one should ask the baby's first name since Nicole and Chad decided not to tell anyone.

My oldest brother walked in the front door and found out his name would be an Uncle. Will had hugs for Chad and Nicole.

Later that evening Will came upstairs to get ready for work and poked his head into my room where I read on my bed. His Rhodesian ridgeback lay curled up beside me. At a hundred and thirty pounds, Archer had become my loyal protector. Will questioned my unhappy face.

I sensed sadness around me even though everything surrounding me was joyous. I desired to be married and have a baby too. Right now, I wasn't sure that would happen. I had a pain in my stomach whenever young adults got a boyfriend, started a killer job, or bought a nice bungalow in the suburbs. I tried to remind myself that eventually marriage and children would fall into place. My goal was to be able to select a picket fence and decide what kind of dog to have with the man of my dreams. I desperately wanted to have Mommy problems. I wished to ask a realtor about school district and busy streets. Should I live in the country or the city? Perhaps somewhere in between would suit me best. Does the house have a pool or hot tub?"

Will craved those things for both of us. He stepped forward to brush away my tear stained cheeks with the pad of his left thumb. I hope Will never stopped calling me Babe. The two of us locked in an embrace we both needed.

Chad phoned early in July to say the baby was a girl. My Mom jumped over the moon with joy. Paint the town pink. In four months I would get to see my niece.

My Mom was anxious to go to the fabric store to look for material for the baby quilt. She and I gathered a list of name guesses from people we knew.

The months ticked by with extreme slowness. I waited patiently to see my niece. Eventually I'd get to meet our newest family member.

August brought extreme heat. It wouldn't be long now, before I could hold my niece in my arms.

I wondered if Chad and Nicole had a name picked out yet. They had some contenders, but nothing permanent. Nicole thought the name Allegra was pretty, but her friend ruined it. Apparently Allegra is the name of an allergy medication. If Chad and Nicole chose to name the baby Allegra, her brother could be named Reactine.

*****

The end of September came when Nicole was due to have the baby. Any time the phone rang in September, my parents ran up in anticipation of the baby coming.

Chad phoned to say the baby would be born within the next few hours. Nicole had gone into labour. He promised he'd call us when we could meet their new baby at the hospital. Until then, my Mother would sew to her heart's content.

In the early hours of September 29th, 2005 my niece was born. Nicole was a champ. We had to go to the hospital to find out her name. We were instructed to bring the list of names people guessed. We had three pages of guesses and nobody hit the correct name.

My parents and I entered Nicole's hospital room. Chad handed our mother her new grand-daughter. Claire had been swaddled. Tears dribbled down my Mom's cheeks. She suited the name perfectly.

My mother suggested Chad and Nicole better not let the other parents see Claire because they'd feel badly their own baby wasn't as beautiful as our baby.

I sat back in a hospital armchair and my Dad passed the baby to me. What a sweetheart. We were going to get along just fine.

Mom & Dad,
I'll go and see the baby later today, after I've had some sleep. I worked last night and I work tonight at the casino.
Will

Later that day Will went to meet his niece with the directions in his hand. Will rounded the corner into the labour and delivery area of the hospital and saw Chad standing in the doorway.

Will was delighted for his brother and sister-in-law. He saw his niece all wrapped up in a pink receiving blanket, laying still in her bassinet. She had just the right combination of both parents. Will lifted her up. Claire fit in his arms because he needed her. Claire left footprints on his heart.

After Will returned home, he walked into the living room to find Dad and I reading and our mother frantically sewing the baby quilt. Will went to see baby because he thought an uncle was expected to do the right thing. He didn't think his emotions to overflow the moment he saw her.

Nicole and Claire came home from the hospital a few days before Thanksgiving. We had pies to order and a meal to plan. We certainly had a lot to be grateful for.

My mother finished sewing the name tag on Claire's quilt the night before Thanksgiving. Nicole eyed each of the pastel fabrics, a work of art. Chad was moved by the beauty of the quilt as a whole. Claire's parents cheered for every smile and coo, even if the movement resulted in a bit of gas.

*****

I turned twenty-three on November 11th 2005. The season's first snow flurries came on my birthday. Claire smiled at my Dad; nobody saw her grin though, so it didn't count.

Claire definitely attached herself to my Dad. From the day she came into the world she had eyes for her Grandpa. She would nuzzle into him and fall fast asleep.

I tired of winter and January had barely begun. Going outside was a pain in the ass. I had warm boots, but it took an engineer to get them on. I preferred early fall.

When Claire came for a visit, she bundled up beyond recognition. Once she was stripped down to her indoor clothes, she was happy to look around. The smiles started as soon as her Grandpa picked her up.

Part of me grew envious of the relationship between Claire and my Dad because my grandfathers never had the opportunity to spend time with me. I wanted closeness with a grandfather, but they had both passed on before I was born. Another part of me was happy to watch my Dad and Claire shine together.

Every time Will held Claire, she cried. I was sure that she would come around. I think she reacted to his loud voice and deep laugh.

When I was little, my Uncle Noah would pick me up and make me laugh. As soon as he opened his mouth and I realized he wasn't my Daddy, tears began. My Dad and his brother looked so much alike that I became mixed-up.

*****

Spring had finally arrived. The crocuses poked through the soil. Will had been seeing someone and he wanted the family to meet her. Love was in the air. Our Mom checked the calendar and chose a date that worked for everyone to have dinner together.

At long last, the appointed date appeared on the calendar. The phone buzzed and Mom let Will and his girlfriend into the building. Claire sat on the play mat with a toy in her hand. Will introduced Julie Chandler before he hung up her coat.

Julie spoke to the adults and stepped into the living room where Claire played. Julie crouched down to her level. Claire looked at Julie and put her arms up to her. Julie bounced up and down with the baby in her arms.

Will couldn't believe what had just transpired. He'd been trying for months to get Claire to let him hold her and Julie picked her up on the first try.

Julie had five nieces and nephews who were all under four, so she was familiar with little ones. Claire touched the lace on Julie's dress and rubbed the texture.

Dear Will,

Julie is a lovely lady and a wonderful fit with our family. I wouldn't say I liked her, if I didn't think she was right for you. I think you complement one another well.

Love,

Megan xo

P.S. I'm pretty sure Nicole thought that Julie was a fantastic person too. She & I aren't easily impressed, so I'd say you should hang onto Julie.

*****

August always made me anxious for back to school whether I returned to school or not. I didn't mind school, but September was typically hot and when they cut the grass my allergies made my nose run. I preferred my air conditioned house. I wouldn't have missed going to school because I valued my social life.

Mom and Dad made a reservation for the family to go out to a nice restaurant for their anniversary. They opted for a beautiful restaurant by a lake. The menu had French words to describe the food.

Perhaps someday I'd have an anniversary to celebrate. Will was the happiest I'd seen him in a long while. He was with the right person for him and they exuded a loving nature when they were together. Chad and Nicole were in a happy place.

We all spoke in unison, "Happy Anniversary Mom and Dad."

As far as I know, the last time my parents had sex was when I was conceived. Why would you mess with the perfection that is me?

At dinner Julie told us that she'd like Will to meet her siblings and their families in Sweden. It meant a big trip, but he was jumping in with both feet. They'd be gone for three and a half weeks.

*****

Scotland was on the way to Sweden, so they stopped for a couple days. Will imagined of playing golf at St. Andrew's for a long time. I wasn't great with geography, but even I knew Scotland was not close to Sweden. Golfing at St. Andrew's was a bucket list item for any golfer worth his salt.

October came and went. Will and Julie had a fabulous time in Sweden seeing the sights and meeting her family.

*****

Now Claire walked on her own two feet. She followed my Dad around the house from room to room. I gave her my best stuff, silly faces and animated storybooks, but Claire didn't pay me much attention. Claire called my Dad "Campy". When Claire couldn't find my Dad she became French. "Ou Campy?" was her favourite question.

*****

Claire was under the impression nobody else could share the same surname as her. Claire called me Auntie Megan. In her two year old mind that was my full name. I spoiled her with cuddles.

One day when Claire was over at our house, my Mom offered to play with bubbles outside, which were always a hit. Claire wanted me to come outside with her, but she knew I couldn't walk. She raised her arms, not knowing what to do next.

Claire understood my illness better than some adults. I've always been in her life, so to Claire my being in a wheelchair was part of her normal. She even copies my exercises whenever she's visiting.

*****

My twenty-fourth birthday came and went. Grey clouds seemed to be occurrence in early November. Will wanted to come over midweek. My Mom and I grew curious as to the reason behind his solo visit. My Dad had a board meeting, but Will decided to come anyway.

Will came in the door with his laptop in hand. When we sat down he appeared to be nervous about something. He had something to show us. Will paused while he booted up his laptop.

We'd already seen the photos from their trip. I hoped he didn't drive all this way to show us a YouTube clip.

Will and Julie brought something back they thought would put us in a cheerful mood. He pulled up a picture of Julie in Scotland. I wrinkled my forehead.

Will showed us an ultrasound picture of a baby and instantly I understood what he meant. They hadn't planned to get pregnant, but Will and Julie were destined to be together forever.

Our Mother put her left arm around Will and squeezed. I stared at the computer screen in shock. "Does everyone but me get to have a baby," I contemplated.

Will and Julie wanted to get married before the baby arrived. The baby was due in the first half of June.

*****

February of 2007 was a dreary month. Will called early one morning, to say the ultrasound showed a baby girl. My Mom could begin to gather the different materials to make another baby quilt.

Will and Julie picked the beginning of March to hold their wedding. My parents and I were excited to be adding to our family.

I thought I'd wear my slate coloured satin dress with the jewels on the top half. I had pewter ballet flats with studs on the toes. I went over my outfit in my mind the night before Will and Julie's wedding.

March 4th arrived and there was a slight chill in the air. I opted to wear my grey Ugg boots, so my legs wouldn't freeze. I brought my ballet flats for the restaurant reception indoors.

The wedding was beautiful. I thought city hall weddings ceremonies could be repetitive all the same, but this lady made my eyes tear up. The justice of the peace spoke of marriage as opposed to a wedding.

Julie, with her kind and gentle soul, meshed well with our family. She and Will moved into an apartment within her parent's home.

Now that the wedding was over, my Mom concentrated on sewing the baby quilt. The crib quilt would be treasured for years to come.

*****

June came and the summer sun shone down. My parents were in baby mode. After supper one evening the phone jingled on the end table. We all tried to grab the phone. Two weeks before the due date Julie had gone into labour.

Shit. The quilt my Mom started wasn't completed. She began a mad scramble to sew.

The baby's birthday was June 3rd, 2007. My parents and I came up to see everyone at the hospital. Will handed the baby to our Mom. He was a proud new father. Zoe was beautiful. My Mom didn't move her gaze off of the baby.

Will passed the baby to Chad. My brothers had glossy eyes at that moment. I held the baby in my arms and took a deep breath of baby lotion.

*****

On the way home from visiting Julie and the baby in the hospital, I rode with Chad. I was happy for Will and Julie, but I wanted to be in love and have a baby someday.

Nicole and Chad went to great lengths to have Claire. I didn't know why getting pregnant came easily for some people and nearly impossible for others.

My Mom laid out the pieces of the baby quilt on the dining room table. My Dad had taken the name tag to be embroidered. You sign a quilt like you do a painting.

Claire met Zoe. She leaned over and kissed her forehead and in her sweet voice she said 'Luff you'.

No one told Will and Julie that Zoe's first poop would come out like toothpaste and resemble roofing tar. Sometimes her poop would look similar to bunny droppings in her diaper. To be fair, neither of them ever asked. The worst parts of having a child were forgotten with a smile or giggle.

Sometime in August of 2007, my Mom finished Zoe's baby quilt, a gorgeous art piece. Will and Julie couldn't speak. The ladybug theme was a perfect idea. The blanket pattern was the same, but made up of totally different fabrics than Claire's quilt.

*****

My parents watched Claire at our house one day in October. She was curious where the baby was. Claire had only seen Zoe at our place, so she thought she lived with us. We told her Zoe was at her house with Uncle Will and Auntie Jules.

"Old MacDonald Had a Farm," streamed through the air from a children's music channel on the television. Claire knew some of the words, so she sang along. Claire continued to sound out words. We didn't always understand her the first time around.

Aside from the usual "Mama and Dada," doll, ball and Campa were some of her favourite words. Oh, and Claire ate goldfish crackers as if they were going out of style.

Claire figured out how we all related to one another. My Dad explained his name was James, but she should call him Grandpa. Somehow she knew her Grandma's name was Rose. Claire wondered why she knew Rose's name and her Grandpa didn't.

Claire went into the living room and began to play with her toys on the mat. Claire told her Grandma her name was Rosalinda. Where did that come from? Don't look at me. I have no clue where she got that name. Google to the rescue. It turns out Rosalinda was the store clerk on a kid's program.

Even as the snow fell outside; the warmth of my family was evident in our demeanor. My whole family was over for dinner. Claire was playing on the red toy mat, introducing Zoe to the farm animals from the barn set. Claire reminded everyone that babies can't talk. Claire was a big girl and Zoe was little.

My parents stood watching their kids and grandkids interact with one another. Life was good. My Dad had said before he had kids of his own, he had three theories for raising children. Now my parents had three offspring and no ideas on child rearing.

*****

The beginning of May started with the sun poking through my shutters. I was going to have a shower; my Mom wheeled me into the bathroom. We babysat Claire that day, so my Mom tried to keep her occupied while I showered. The bathroom was laid out by an occupational therapist and tweaked by a mobility specialist to suit all of my needs.

Claire squeezed herself into the bathroom to know what I was doing. I informed her I cleaned up. She offered to help. I think she had to see how I showered because I can't walk. My Mom escorted her to the living room where an assortment of toys to play with and books to read awaited her.

June had settled in and Zoe came over with her parents. Zoe pointed at the little ball that lay still on the dark hardwood floor of the living room. Julie pointed and Zoe stood and then sat down to crawl after the ball.

The next time we saw Zoe, she'd be on her feet. My parents pondered the thought as they waved goodbye from the balcony.

*****

Summer came to an end. We squeezed the last bit of the August heat like a tube of toothpaste that neared empty. Will anxiously hung around to find out what we would think if they had another baby. I wasn't sure where he was going with his line of questioning.

As it turns out, they hoped to have another baby. Will held Julie's hand next to his heart. "That's wonderful news," I exclaimed. Somehow, I was emotional at the possibility of me not becoming a parent, single or otherwise.

Of course I'd be thrilled if and when Will and Julie added more to their. My parents were marvelous grandparents. My Father stretched his arms out to Zoe and plucked her up from the mat where she tried to crawl. I suppose having no kids meant when the kids got crabby or had a bad odor coming from a diaper, I could send them back to their parents.

Thanksgiving preparations had begun. The smells of fall: brush burning, pumpkin pie, maple syrup, cinnamon and fresh apples lingered in the air.

Dessert was 'Pavlova'; a hard meringue layered with Devon cream and topped with fresh berries and whipping cream. The taste was heavenly in my opinion. The Devon cream was rich, but the rest of the dessert went down easy after a heavy dinner.

Will inquired as to when babies generally stopped wearing diapers. Will didn't have any idea what answer he'd get.

"It depends on the child, but usually between two and three years old." My Mother shook her head. Will had been three years and one month when he was fully potty-trained.

Apparently Will missed that day in prenatal class. A lot of shitty diapers had been changed since he attended Lamaze class. He couldn't be expected to retain all of the pre-baby information.

*****

The first month of my 2009 Golden Retriever calendar was ultra-cute. How could they miss with fluffy puppies? My family had grown up with dogs around. Big dogs didn't scare me; they kept me warm at night.

Will and Julie added one more to their family. He or she would be born in July, but they could make their appearance early. Two kids and a dog, they were living the American dream, in Canada. I was happy for them. I wished I had positive news to share with my family. Viewing Law & Order with my parents didn't qualify as an announcement.

*****

The following month brought more snow. The pure white snow draped the town in sparkle before streets became a brown slushy mess within hours.

Chad was over to pick up Claire. She ran into her Dad's waiting arms. She had been excellent. I now had an excuse to watch Disney movies. Chad went to talk with our Dad while Claire continued to play.

I heard Claire whining for my Mom, but we were in the midst of a conversation. My Mom held up her hand to get her to remain quiet until we finished talking.

Claire grew more agitated. She thought didn't hear her. We watched as she continued to draw our attention to herself. She pointed to her eyes to get my Mom to make eye contact. Then she gestured to her whole face. "See my eyes, look at my face. Now listen." I found the situation funny, but I couldn't laugh.

One of Claire's teachers would use the words to get a misbehaving child to focus on them.

Claire tested her boundaries. She didn't make the rules, the adults in her life did. When someone spoke, she had to wait until they ended before speaking.

*****

March was the month Will and Julie could find out whether they would be having a boy or girl. My Mom and I couldn't wait to find out the sex of the new baby. My Dad was curious, but he went about making his coffee and reading the local newspaper.

Hi Everyone.

We're having a boy.
That's one of every kind they make, so our family is complete.
Lots of love,
Will, Julie, Big Sister Zoe, Archer xo xo xo xo

I intended to go shopping for boy toys and clothes. Somehow my Dad knew that was coming and rolled his blue eyes to the sky.

My Mom had to pick out the main fabric for the baby boy's quilt. I liked the farm animal theme. I sat among pretty bolts of fabric while my mother perused the rest of the fabric store.

April was getting closer. Most of the clothing stores had a selection of Easter dresses and outfits on display. I adored a plaid shirt on a baby boy. Some of the outfits were mini versions of adult clothing.

I browsed the newborn section of Baby Gap with my best friend Olivia in. We were in a baby store so it wasn't unusual to see pregnant women. Olivia held up a cherry pink bathing suit with a ruffled top. I had one just like that when I was small. Oddly enough, Liv had a similar swimsuit when she was a toddler.

*****

July was still a few days away, but the baby had dropped and could make his first appearance at any moment. We were all on high alert. I couldn't concentrate on mindless television entertainment.

Text From: Will McIntyre
Julie is in labour. xo
Reply:
Thanks for the update.
Keep us posted.
Love,
Auntie Megan xo

When the baby was born, my brother phoned. His son was named Liam Ryan McIntyre and he was adorable. My Dad could add another person to our family tree.

If Liam had not come out of Julie, she'd have doubts about whether he belonged to her. He didn't look much like her at all. Julie cuddled her baby boy skin to skin. He had the McCheeks.

*****

During late July, my Mom had Liam's baby quilt for Will and Julie to open. Liam was five weeks early, so technically the gift was on time.

Will and Julie had wondered about the colour scheme of the quilt for some time. The blanket was stunning. Julie held it up and admired the fabric and the farm themed wall hanging. Will kissed his mother's cheek.

I was fond of the traditions my family had. Maybe someday my Mom would make a quilt for my offspring. Then again, maybe kids aren't in the cards for me. My happiness didn't rely on me someday having children, but I found it hard to give up on parenthood.

Being an Auntie to three beautiful children meant the world to me. My face lights up when the opportunity to read to each of them arises. I soaked up all of the cuddles, and hugs. When they cried, my heart hurt.

*****

I am proud of myself and deserve all of the accolades I've been given all day. I never imagined my university career would take so long, but in the end my degree has the same value as someone who finished on time.

Changes

Oh come on. I'm hungry. I tried to listen to the speaker, but she was rather wordy. I had to learn to be patient. Breathe.

*****

I turned eighteen when I went to live in residence for university. I was an adult on paper sure, but after I moved home, I felt like a bigger adult. Although I came home quite a bit on weekends, I learned to do some laundry on my own. I'd formed friendships that would last forever.

The following school year, I lived at home and got dropped off or rode to school with Liv. I liked living at home, but I missed the life on-campus and the variety of food in the cafeteria.

*****

In my second year, I was required to take statistical psychology even though I knew that I'd never use this in the future. Math was far from my favourite. I didn't understand why. I was curious to know who made up the formula and why they did. Or how did the author of each equation know that it would work out each time?

Morgan was in my lecture, so we decided to pick a day each week to work on our stats homework at my house. I don't know if I would've done as well without being able to talk the answers out with her.

Morgan was living off campus during our second year of university, so my mother invited her to stay for dinner after our homework was finished. Morgan always accepted with a grin stretching across her face. My Mom wanted her to have a home cooked meal even though she was away from her family. My Mom would pack up some leftover food for Morgan to have another meal at her apartment.

On some days when Morgan and I were doing our stats homework,

Nicole would drop off leftovers for us to eat while we finished our math. We munched on pretzels and cheesies. Hence, our formula notebooks had orange dust on the edges of some pages.

You never knew who was coming to dinner. There was never a shortage of food around our house. Sometimes Chad and Nicole dropped by on the way to her parents for dinner. Morgan was a member of our family while she was over.

*****

When Morgan met her future husband, she brought him for dinner at our house while he visited. My Mom made baked ziti. We're not Italian, but they talked about ziti on some dramas. We looked up a recipe and a classic was born.

Morgan and her boyfriend Felix Westin were adorable together. Months passed and Felix was back at his university. While we were doing our statistics homework one Friday, Morgan mentioned that if she and Felix were to have a daughter someday she'd like to call her Vivi Jane. Morgan and Felix's relationship was moving fast. I knew that they were serious, but discussing baby names was a step further. But I guess when you're in love, why wait?

The following Christmas Felix worked with Morgan's father to make her proposal story special. Dr. Baxter did photography as a hobby, so he snapped a picture of Felix's hands holding the ring box open. Felix wrapped the matted frame in a pyjama box to throw Morgan off. Felix handed her the box and as she removed the tissue he got down on one knee.

Dr. Baxter captured many memories over the years, so Morgan and her Mom Colleen weren't suspicious when he got closer to create an accurate reaction from the girls. Ladies were keen on the story. Guys are either irritated that they didn't think of the idea, or pressured into making their engagement equally spectacular.

*****

In front of about a hundred and twenty people at their church in Kitchener, Felix Westin and Morgan Baxter sealed their marriage vows with a kiss. The reception was at a large banquet hall done up in teal, brown, and orange to look like a Caribbean sunset.

*****

My parents went to Wales to visit my mother's pen pal Rebecca and her husband Ethan Kellingston. They'd been writing since they were ten years old and that year Rebecca and my Mom would turn sixty. I was still on my feet and my brothers dropped in for an overnight, so I wasn't alone for the full two weeks. I had a group of friends that my parents trusted.

One night while my parents were gone a bunch of my friends went to a local pub. We walked out with our arms linked. Jonah declared he was staying over at my place. I already knew that we were all going to sleep at my house, but Jonah was loud for the benefit of some people he worked with. I was secretly thrilled that I was with the cool kids.

So we all went back to my house and got out the sleeping bags and blankets to spread around the family room. Lassie settled on the tile floor by the back door. I grabbed some extra pillows and made my bed before I closed my eyes for the night.

I remember hearing the phone ring, but I figured I'd let the answering machine get the call. The phone kept ringing. After five rings, the noise went silent. I was happy to not have to deal with phone calls this early in the morning. Then I heard Jonah talking. Oh shit. My Aunt Nina and Uncle Russell were headed up north and they decided to phone me. Jonah explained that they didn't have the wrong number. By that time I eagerly awaited for him to hand me the phone.

I worried how my Aunt and Uncle would perceive the situation. I was an adult and I didn't have an orgy. I had a co-ed sleepover and my parents knew what was happening while they were on vacation. Jonah was my friend and the rest wasn't anybody else's business.

*****

Megan,
Guess what the attached photo is of? … Times up.
Felix and I are pregnant. I'm 3½ months along. We're thrilled to be able to tell our family and friends.
Morgan xo

My life was becoming full of babies and toddlers. Being an Auntie is a privilege I don't take for granted, but I still longed for a baby to call my own. With a boyfriend in sight and the list of prospective male suitors getting smaller by the day, I wasn't likely to be a mother.

Morgan,
What fabulous news. I'm ecstatic for you & Felix.
Your parents must be over the moon about becoming Grandparents.
Hugs & kisses for your family.
Megan

Morgan and Felix weren't going to find out the sex of the baby, which made waiting all the more difficult. How do you buy clothes for a baby you don't know the sex of? When the time comes the doctor would announce whether they have a girl or boy.

Felix and Morgan's due date came and went and still no action. Four days passed and her water broke at five in the morning. Several hours passed and still no babe. Finally at just after noon a baby girl was born. Vivi Jane Westin was a beautiful addition to the Westin family.

We drove to Morgan's parents' home for lunch and to meet the precious baby girl. The food was delicious and the company was great. I brought the smallest Brock hoodie I could find. Vivi wouldn't fit the sweatshirt until she was a toddler, but I couldn't resist Brock clothing on children.

*****

I grew up in a four level side-split, located on a deep lot within a large crescent in Niagara Falls. We had wonderful neighbours, a big yard, a swimming pool, a fire pit and our own slice of nature in the city.

In the wintertime, the plows would make a pile of snow on the center median and all of the neighbourhood children would put on their winter gear and head out to play. We would build forts and slides and play for hours on end. Afterwards I went home and my Mom made me hot chocolate while I took off my snowsuit.

Our neighbours mostly stayed the same, aside from the odd move. During the summer months, we had a block party in the middle of the crescent. Every household brought a dish to share. The adults talked and the little kids played. Zack brought out a game similar to corn hole. Zack's game was one he crafted out of two sheets of plywood and some old beanbags. He called the game 'Puck Off'. We were lucky none of the children had a speech impediment.

During my childhood, I made a lot of memories. I was the only girl in a crescent full of boys, so we played a lot of sports. The fact that I got so much exercise as a kid probably aided me in my search for balance.

I do remember playing cops and robbers in a friend's unfinished basement. The stairs had open risers and we made that the jail. The only way in was through the small opening in the stairs and most of the kids could fit between the stair boards.

A few years later, I was over to the same house to feed the dog while the family was out for the day. The basement had been finished and the stairs had been filled in. I stared at the spot where I once slipped through as a child and my jaw dropped in shock at how small the risers were. There was no denying that I was a skinny child, but I wasn't the only scrawny pre-teen hanging out on the crescent.

*****

There was a scary time in my life. In the fall of 2007 my Mom became sick. Our family doctor ran tests to eliminate certain illnesses. My Mom developed a deep cough and at times she couldn't talk. My Mom called her Mother each night after dinner was completed. When she had a coughing spell, I would take the phone and finish her phone call.

One night we had been for dinner at my Auntie Leona and Uncle Ted's home. We were all concerned about my mother's health. She had a late morning appointment with our family doctor the next morning to get some test results.

On the way back to Niagara my Mom started coughing and couldn't seem to catch her breath. My Dad pulled over and assessed the situation. My Mother had to go to the nearest hospital. I was to phone my brother Will and have him pick me up at the hospital. This was before texting was all the rage, so I dialed Will's cell phone. I heard his voice, but when I opened my mouth no sound came out. My Dad took the phone and relayed the message.

Will met us at the hospital and I went home with him. We went through a drive-thru for some hot apple cider. The warm drink was somewhat calming as Will drove toward home. The whole family was worried.

I had to call and cancel a breakfast date my parents had with another couple early the next morning. My plan was to be vague, so I didn't stress them out unnecessarily, because at that point all we could do was speculate.

I remember my parents coming home that night and thinking about what was wrong. The doctors at the hospital didn't drop the bomb, but they were suspicious about cancer. The dreaded 'c word' could be why my mother was sick. Nobody wants to hear their own name and cancer in the same sentence.

The next day my Dad entered my room and nodded, indicating that my Mom had cancer. She had a biopsy between Christmas and New Year's. Olivia's Mom phoned to make sure that my Mother had the best care at the hospital where she was a nurse.

The biopsy results showed that my Mother had lymphoma. One month after a diagnosis of cancer, my parents were waiting in the lymphoma clinic reception area. That day my Mother started the first of six rounds of chemotherapy. The plan was to obliterate the tumor that was pressing on her lungs causing her to cough.

I was at home that day, so Olivia came over with some fast food to distract my mind. We didn't talk about my Mom because we both would have ended up bawling. I was happy to have company on such a tense day.

My parents came home with books and pages of literature about lymphoma and where to go to get a wig. The nurse practitioner had indicated that her hair would fall out around her second chemotherapy treatment. Rather than have your hair fall out in the butter dish while making toast, she suggested that my Mom just buzz the hair after a clump came loose.

The wig hairdresser saw my Mom's natural style and came so close that some people didn't realize that it wasn't her own hair. My mother and I always pointed out hair pieces to each other, so we were both glad she didn't have a wig that was obviously not her hair.

My Mom was nervous about wearing her wig out in public. When my parents picked up the wig my mother's hair hadn't started to fall out, but she wore it home. My parents made a quick run into Costco. None of the other shoppers gave her an odd look. The employee thought that the photo and the lady in front of him, matched.

After they returned home, my Mom lost her first lump of her own hair. My Dad buzzed her hair over the bathroom sink. My Mother had the same head as her grandfather. She never let us see her bald head, she always had a scarf or winter hat on when she was around me.

If you had to get cancer, the kind of lymphoma was more treatable than others. Aside from the original biopsy it wouldn't be necessary for my Mother to have surgery. That was a huge weight lifted off her shoulders.

Our family banded together in stressful times. When my hair got longer than what was in style, Chad went with me. Nicole and I went to a nearby restaurant and had a feast of appetizers. Will stayed home a lot to spend time with me and be with our Mother.

I don't remember a lot during this time period of time. I think I blocked the thoughts about my Mother being sick because I felt so helpless because there was nothing I could do to make her well again. My family tried to be optimistic that our Mom would be better after her treatments were over with.

Cancer is never a good word to hear. I think as a family we drew closer to each other. We all huddled together to protect our beloved Mother.

None of us had a magic pill to make her better, so we all pitched in and did what we could around the house. Will would make dinner on some nights. My Dad did the laundry. Chad or Nicole would run errands for the family and make sure I had what I needed.

Although I couldn't do a lot of household chores, I could wipe the bathroom counter and clean the sink after a day of use.

When my Mother had finished six chemotherapy appointments, she had a CAT scan to see how much the drugs had shrunk the tumor. If the tumor was still there, the doctors had the option of adding more chemo treatments. My Mom was nervous because her energy was already depleted. She didn't know if she could handle more of the drugs.

Luckily the tumor had shrunk enough, so extra chemo wasn't needed. After a few weeks her hair would start to slowly grow back. My Mom's stamina was low and would be next to nothing for the next six months.

*****

Our home was becoming too much for my parents to take care of without help, so they signed up for a lawn care service. The fact that I couldn't get to different rooms without using stairs, meant our house was working against us.

My parents and I began searching for condos in our area. There was the bungalow condo and the high rise condo. I was partial to the bungalow style condo, but my parents wanted a high rise style with underground parking.

We didn't even look at bungalow condos with an attached garage, which bothered me in the beginning. I realize that my parents were using their own money, but they didn't have to rub it in by totally ignoring my preferences. I know that I might never get to own a home, so I would've liked to have put my two cents in.

We toured a unit in Niagara Falls and I saw that high rise condos weren't all bad. In fact, I knew that I could live in a vertical subdivision.

Over the next year we saw units at high rise condominiums throughout the Niagara Region and Hamilton. There was an address that we liked in the Falls.

We looked in Stoney Creek because my brother and sister-in-law lived nearby in a neighboring townhouse. They didn't mind us living nearby because the townhouse that they lived in was likely not their final home. None of us were expecting to be amazed by every inch of what we saw outside. The grounds were impeccable. We stepped into the lobby of what is now our home and fell further love with our surroundings.

*****

My family began to pare down our belongings and clear out our basement to get ready for a garage sale. Some stuff I was fine to let go of, but I found it hard to let go of my bar fridge. I used the fridge when I was in residence. After I moved home, the fridge went to our family room in our make shift bar zone. When a lady came to the garage sale and offered sixty dollars for the spotless fridge it eased the stress of thinning out our possessions.

At our garage sale, our neighbours donated their time and goods to sell. I sat in a lawn chair at the mouth of our garage. Rich Dolen sat nearby. He lived across the street from us with his wife Vanessa and their three year old daughter named Bailey.

Our neighbour Zack came over to donate a set of golf clubs, but instead he bought my Dad's set of clubs and bag. His wife Mia was out for the day, so my parents joked that Zack wasn't allowed to buy décor items without written consent. Zack did buy a series of plates with grapes on them that he thought Mia would like. When the garage sale was over, Zack was our best customer.

To get our home ready for sale, everyone pitched in. My parents had to replace the drain in the main bathroom. I was vaguely aware of what was going on upstairs. I was reading on the sofa in our living room. That was until I heard my parents speak.

"Slide it in gently."

"Ouch."

"Pull out quickly."

"Let's try this again."

"Aim the long part on a downward angle."

"That's better. Can you spin it around a bit?"

"Pull it tight and then release it."

"Harder."

"Ahh. That's the way to do it."

I trusted that they were plumbing. Otherwise, I don't expect my parents would ever bring the topic of sex in our bathroom up for discussion.

When our basement was empty but for a few clear plastic bins, my parents found a realtor and signed on to sell our house. I don't care how old you are, seeing a "for sale" sign on the front lawn of the house you grew up in wasn't easy. My entire family knew that moving was the right thing to do at the time, but seeing a for sale sign up made my eyes fill with tears.

Our neighbours weren't eager to see us leave. Zack and Mia, along with Rich and Vanessa, were not prepared for us to move thirty-five minutes away from them. At that point, we hadn't bought a condo yet. I had become friends with Vanessa and was used to seeing her nearly every day. We would congregate on our front deck and talk about our day. Once we moved life would be different, no matter where we ended up.

There were several showings a day after my parents had made the deal with the realtor, Thomas Huberto. This was a good sign that the house was priced to sell. A bidding war was too much to expect. A day later, Thomas had an offer of nearly full price. My parents talked it over and accepted the deal.

*****

Now we had to find a new place to live. We looked online to see what was for sale at the condominium we were partial to in Niagara Falls. The only unit available was a one bedroom and I didn't believe my parents fancied sleeping on a pull out couch in the living room.

My parents made contact with the realtor that had shown us a few condos the year before. Gary Olette met us at the condominium near Lake Ontario the following afternoon. He was able to get us in to see seven units.

When we entered the unit that we later bought; we were amazed by the view of the water and the escarpment. The layout was perfect for us. There were three bedrooms to the right and the living space to the left.

My Mom liked the size of the balcony. The hardwood throughout for accessibility was fantastic for my mobility. My Dad was enamored with the floor to ceiling windows off of the family room. My Mom had admired white shutters in other people's houses. Every room had the white shutters. Around each corner, there was a feature that made us excited about the possibility of living in that very unit.

Gary wrote up an offer and submitted it to the other realtor. The two debated back and forth until all of the parties involved were satisfied. The deal was signed the following morning and we had officially bought a condo. The closing date was less than a month away.

Our neighbours were happy for us, but they weren't sure moving to a new city was going to work out. Time would tell. Zack and Mia had a moving barbeque in our honour.

*****

My Aunt Lily had a new gentleman friend that she'd being seeing for a while now. She had the extended family to meet him. His name was Martin Preston. He brought a lot of light to my Aunt's life.

Martin gave the best hugs around. He wasn't trying to impress anyone; he was just a natural fit in our family. Martin connected well with every aspect of my Aunt's social circles.

My Aunt Lily golfed at a local club and so did Martin. They each had family that was spread out, so they travelled together. My Aunt Lily was a long time resident of Georgetown and so was Martin, so they each had friends within the city.

*****

Morgan had sent me a photo of a loaf of bread in her oven. I didn't know what she meant by the bread. I peered at the picture and an instant later I knew that it was a riddle for a bun in the oven. Vivi was going to be a big sister.

Six months passed and baby Marco Owen Westin was born. The Westin's were now a family of four. When Marco was three months old we visited them in their forever home.

Vivi Jane was now three and a half years old. She showed me her collection of books and introduced me to her new brother. The home was a two-story, so while my parents went on a tour of the upstairs Vivi took me on a video tour using her iPad.

*****

Will and Julie dreamed of raising their family up north or in farm country. They wished to live in a small town, where everyone knew each other and looked out for the kids as if they were their own children.

. All this talk about a new residence got Will and Julie thinking about their own possible move. My brother and sister-in-law lived with Julie's parents. Having four adults in the house meant that child care wasn't an issue. Daycare costs were the equivalent of a car payment for some families.

Will and Julie had some money set aside to make a down payment on a house, but they weren't sure which town to live in yet. Living near Toronto wasn't high on Will's list and Julie had a similar opinion.

A couple of weeks went by and my parents got the keys to our new home. The movers arrived as my Mom and I backed out of the driveway. I didn't want to see the truck being loaded. We passed Rich and Vanessa who were watching Bailey ride her pink tricycle on the sidewalk. Tears stung my eyes and rolled down my cheeks.

I went to my brother and sister-in-law's home, only a ten minute walk from our new condo. I knew that I couldn't do much but get in the way. I woke up in my bed at our former home and would go to sleep in my bed at the condo. The miracle of having movers worked in our favour.

When I arrived at the condo later that night, the mover's had hung our artwork on the hooks that the previous owner had used. Some of their choices worked while others were just meant to get the paintings off of the floor.

My Mom and Nicole made my bed and placed a new duvet cover I had picked out for my new room. I realized I should go with a quilt when I got new bedding. It takes a lot of effort to shake the duvet into the case.

About a week after we settled into our new place, Rich and Vanessa came over to see us. They were amazed by the space and were quite taken with the view. Bailey sat on the couch next to me doodling on a sketch pad.

The weather happened to be stinking hot when they got there. Each unit has control over the temperature in their space. My Mom had the air conditioning on and the air was cool. Rich wondered if we were hanging meat in the kitchen. He wasn't used to the air conditioning being set so low and wasn't reluctant about speaking his mind.

*****

Chad and Nicole were looking for their forever home, but hadn't found what they were looking for. Nicole was keen on a house that didn't require too much work in order to move in. Chad hoped they could find a house that had little projects he could take his time completing.

Being close to my brother and sister-in-law allowed us to be more social with them. We sometimes went for walks around the block with Chad and Nicole. My parents and I got to know our new neighbourhood along the way. We got to know the dogs that were friendly and the owners who didn't speak.

I liked having a relative in the same city. My parents learned which grocery store to go to for fresh fruit and vegetables and which drugstore carried the brands we liked. My brother pointed out which farmer's market to go to and where to buy great meat that didn't cost an arm and a leg.

Our extended family was that much closer since we moved to the condo. Auntie Leona and Uncle Ted were now under seventeen minutes from our front door to theirs.

Daphne lived in Grimsby. We were practically neighbours now. This was fabulous because now we could have hot chocolate or a tea and discuss what was new.

Daphne had been dating the same guy since just after we met. The way she spoke of Jason Yaughters sounded like they'd be headed down the proverbial aisle within the next couple of years.

The choice to move was hard. Once we made the decision on where we were going and what type of accommodation we wanted, every detail seemed to fall into place. Moving is never easy, whether you've stayed in one place for a long time or pack up your belongings every few years. We were where we were supposed to be.

Stoney Creek was roughly halfway between Niagara and Toronto depending on where in the city you were going. That meant that we could maintain our friendships in Niagara Falls and still be close to events in Toronto.

Life constantly changes. Growing-up, our front door should have been a revolving door. Someone was on their way to or from work seemingly all the time.

*****

Hi Megan.

I'm still on vacation and having fun. While we were touring, I found a cute café that offered free wireless internet, so I took the opportunity to write to you. Eric proposed. I'm over the moon. I have told some family, but I'll wait to tell everyone else once we arrive home. I know an engagement isn't official until you change your status on social media, but I'll do that once I tell all of my extended family.

I'm not one to brag, but the ring is gorgeous. I can't wait to show you in person.

Liv xo

*****

Chad and Nicole walked over to our new home with Claire tucked into her stroller. They had been looking online and found a house listing that they both adored.

My parents and I cared for Claire while Chad and Nicole toured the house in person with their realtor. When they returned their faces were filled with joy mixed with apprehension. Chad and Nicole had submitted an offer to buy their dream home.

After back and forth banter between realtors, the house belonged to Chad and Nicole. Chad and Nicole could move into their new home in the middle of summer. Instead of living a ten minute walk from where my parents and I lived, Chad and Nicole were a ten minute car ride in the next town over.

Grimsby had a small town ambiance with amenities close by. Chad and Nicole's two-story home was out of a fairy tale. There's a step at the front door, but Chad and our Dad can get me into the main level without too much trouble.

Nicole was comfortable in the kitchen. She liked to cook and see people enjoy their meal. I sampled Nicole's baking from time to time and was never disappointed. Her cheesecake doesn't require the use of an oven and the dessert was bar none, the best I'd ever eaten.

Chad and Will both had summer jobs at an Italian restaurant, so they learned to make sauce and fresh pasta. Chad was glad when spring arrived because he could dust off their barbeque and grill vegetables and meat.

*****

Megan,
Would you like to meet at the movie theatre up on the mountain?
Maybe we can see a comedy.
I'll pick you up. Your condo is on the way to the theatre. On Saturday we
could go to a matinee. I'll pick you up at your place around noon.
Daphne

I was glad to go to the movies. I always had a good time, but didn't often see a show at the theatre.

Daphne stared at my wheelchair. In her head she formulated a checklist. As she wrestled with the chair, I neglected to tell her the footrests detached from the frame of the chair in order to fit in the back of the car. Oops.

*****

Liv and Eric wished to have their wedding and reception all at one location. They settled on a venue with a beautiful garden area that would hold the ceremony and a large room with French doors to the courtyard. There was also a hotel attached to the location for out of town guests.

Ten months later, Eric and Olivia tied the knot in front of about sixty-five family members and friends. The sun was shining down on the minister and the joyful couple.

For my birthday, Liv had a professional photographer's picture from her wedding framed for me. My niece Claire thought the photo of me with my Mommy and Daddy was cute. The photo was of Olivia and Eric, with me in the middle. In her mind, pictures with three people were automatically parents and their child.

*****

Daphne and I went out to a desserts only restaurant. I have a sweet tooth. I know sugar isn't healthy, but I don't eat dessert every day. Once in a while, I crave a fuzzy peach or a piece of key lime pie.

Daphne and I got caught up on boyfriends, or in my case the lack thereof. Her sister and brother-in-law had a baby girl about the same time as Nicole had Claire. Hearing the word Auntie and your own name was cool. Her niece is named Lucy.

We'd been chatting for a while when I caught sight of her ring finger.

154

I paused and she nodded. Daphne and I hugged as our desserts arrived. What perfect timing. She was keen on my parents and I being there on her and Jason's big day.

A few weeks later I met Daphne & Jason at Memphis Fire Barbeque Company, for dinner. The restaurant staff knew my name. The hostess gathered the menus and showed us to our table. Pete often waited. I always ordered a Cherry Coke.

We all loved barbequed food and their super creamy macaroni and cheese. Pulled pork and cheese burgers graced our plates, but not for long. Seriously, if you haven't been, go early and come hungry.

*****

Liv and I met for an afternoon of shopping on a Friday in late March. When we arrived my parents and I sat down in the food court area. I could smell the burgers and poutine from across the room.

Olivia came in the automatic sliding doors wearing a flowing top, but it was nothing out of the ordinary for her wardrobe. She asked if we minded getting a bite to eat before we shopped. I was all for that idea because my mouth was watering.

Olivia pulled out a sheet with a little Blip on the paper. Eric and Liv affectionately referred to the baby as Blip. Until they knew the sex of the baby they would toss around name ideas. Olivia was fond of Bianca for a girl, while Eric liked Alexandra.

Five months later out popped a baby boy. Liv had a new respect for labour and delivery nurses. They put up with a lot of shit, literally and figuratively. The pregnant lady was free to unearth her pain and emotion on anybody in the delivery suite. Once the baby emerged, all was forgiven. Watching a family grow by two itty bitty feet makes everything worthwhile in the end. Chase Eric Dickerson was a handsome little guy.

*****

Will and Julie became quite fond of the town of Napanee, Ontario. One of Will's best friends, Nathaniel Laughlin, grew-up in a neighbouring crossroads. Julie became good friends with Nathaniel's wife Emily, so they wouldn't be moving to a new area not knowing anybody.

The town of Napanee was large enough to have convenience stores, excellent schools, a splash pad for the kids, a library, several restaurants, a movie theatre and plenty of nature all around. The air seemed cleaner than Toronto or any city within the Greater Toronto Area.

A house that was accessible for me was high on Will and Julie's list. That way I could come and visit and stay for three or four days. The kids could show me their rooms and I could read them bedtime stories.

Julie found work in Napanee doing accounting for a major drug manufacturing company. Soon after, Will was offered a job as a manager of security for the same employer.

After working with a realtor and touring dozens of houses, they opened the door to what would end up being their home. It was a ranch style bungalow with a basement and it fit the needs of everyone. The lot was a half-acre of a picturesque nature setting, right on the Napanee River.

Although Zoe wasn't born in Napanee, she did her best to get there as soon as she could. Zoe liked dress-up and princesses much like other four year old girls, but she also played outside in the dirt. Zoe was delighted to play with boys. I saw her blossoming from a quiet toddler into a young girl. I'd forgotten how many questions kids ask, like: "Why? Do you sleep all day? What is a moment?"

Liam was still a toddler and was happy wherever you put him. He was hyper aware of the people around him. As long as he could see one of his people, he would be totally peaceful. The moment he lost sight of Mommy or Daddy, he started to become upset. All babies seem to go through a phase where they have to be near their parents.

*****

Daphne and Jason chose to have their wedding in the distillery district of Toronto. The ceremony space was inside an old distillery. We weren't in Kansas anymore. The setting was in a high end part of the city. On a long weekend in October my parents and I were among the invited guests at Daphne and Jason's wedding.

I was fond of non-traditional weddings. I adored it when brides and grooms aren't afraid to tie the knot the way they saw fit. A wedding should be an expression of the couple, and the lovebirds should decide whether that means being in a church or under the stars.

*****

I truly believe someone was looking out for us when we moved. Living in our chosen condo building has been excellent for all of us. To protect our investment, my Dad joined the board of directors. Having the kitchen, living area, washroom and bedrooms on one floor was ideal for me. Being close to her oncologist allowed my Mom to relax a little.

I have a longer list of why I'm on cloud nine living in Stoney Creek. I am thrilled to be closer to my neuromuscular doctor and cardiologist. I'm under the care of doctors with résumés that stretch around the world. I know that the average person might not understand why I'm blessed to have these doctors in my life. I am lucky to have such a comprehensive medical team. At no point in time have I ever been treated as a number.

*****

I am fortunate to live in the same building as a published author, Ben Guyatt. I didn't seek out his guidance; he offered his assistance in getting me into writing. Ben was a source of encouragement. He believed in me and I started to have faith that I could do anything I set my mind to. Maybe I wasn't going to ever run a marathon, but you get the idea. Ben knew my father from being on the board of directors of our condo building.

Ben did a monthly column for a local newspaper and he wanted to write about me. At first, I thought I didn't want to have my story plastered on any media platform. After I gave the offer some thought, I agreed to be interviewed for the column. I was really nervous as I'd never done anything that opened me up to so many people.

I completed the talk with Ben, but not without shedding a few tears. I figured if I did the interview, I had to be as raw as possible for to it to be a successful column. I thought the conversation went as well as was possible.

When the paper came out, part of me hoped the readers liked the article. Another part of me was nervous for me to be content with the column. To this day, whenever I read the paper my eyes water because I'm happy. Ben nailed the impression of me, right down to the core.

From that moment on, I was a new person. I could open myself up a lot easier than was once possible. If somebody didn't appreciate my disability, then they were probably not worth my time to begin with. Life is a continual sorting process.

*****

Over the course of a couple years, I became good friends with Ben.

157

I think our friendship was one of mutual admiration and respect for one another. We can have a conversation about any topic currently nagging one of us and know whatever was said would stay between us.

I was never one that longed to be the center of attention and that was still true. I learned that I shouldn't hide because of my disability. I didn't have to wear layers to conceal my back scar. Now I put on a hoodie because I was cold and not because I hoped to remain hidden.

*****

My cousin Norah was getting married on the weekend, so I was anxious to look and feel my best. Exercise was a big part of feeling well. I was an honorary bridesmaid, whatever that encompassed. I guess I'd find out on the wedding day because nobody I questioned seemed to know either.

Norah and her fiancé got married in the conservatory of an old castle in Toronto. The late afternoon wedding meant the guests could have cocktails on the large outdoor patio. Later we watched the sunset over Lake Ontario.

The day was beautiful, although I still wasn't sure what the definition of an honorary bridesmaid was. I got my makeup done with the other girls and handed out programs to arriving guests. I didn't have to walk down an aisle for which I was grateful because I didn't like going through the middle of a crowd.

Norah and I were connected to each other because we wanted to be. At the end of the day we were best friends.

*****

Shortly after Norah and Lucas returned from their honeymoon, they announced that they were pregnant. The whole family was excited to have a new baby to cuddle.

*****

I met Daphne at the mall one Saturday in January for lunch at one of our favourite spots. The restaurant served deep fried pickles. I wasn't pregnant, but I still craved pickles.

Before my parents went for lunch elsewhere in the shopping center, Daphne handed the three of us a paper from the ultra sound. I peered at her and she pulled her shirt tight so we could see her baby bump.

Now we had an excuse to order deep fried pickles with a side of deep fried pickles. I was happy for Jason and Daphne. They were overjoyed at the news of the upcoming baby.

Daphne and Jason didn't wish to find out the sex of the baby before the birth. Daphne had talked her sister into being surprised in the delivery room. Daphne was curious, but she didn't peek at her ultrasound file.

Megan.
We had a boy. His name is Cohen Blake Yaughters. I cannot wait for you to meet him.
He was 7 lbs. at birth and yes the birth was painful, but so worth the effort in the end.
Daphne

*****

Nine months from the date of Lucas and Norah's wedding, baby Helena Lane was born. What a sweet disposition Helena had. Unfortunately the marriage didn't last. Having Helena gave Norah a new sense of purpose.

*****

The year I was born, my family got a "Commodore 64". That model of computer would probably be worth a bit of money if we still had it. So, computers have always been a part of my life. When I was in my late teens, I had to use the computer a lot for my school work, so my parents got me my own desktop computer. Sometime in my twenties, I switched from a desktop to a laptop computer.

Now I can get email and monitor my social media accounts in the palm of my hand on a cell phone or tablet. Information is so easily obtained by using simple search terms. There are cell phones that let you speak the question and give the answer orally.

I can do shopping online and the parcel arrives at my door. I can listen to music while I surf the web. The laptop makes so much possible. I can check my bank account or buy a book.

I use my laptop to write while listening to the same song on repeat. Music provides just enough distraction. I prefer to have a consistent routine and get into a writing rhythm. Sometimes I pop in a piece of gum for an added beat.

*****

My parents and I made our first of many trips to Napanee about six weeks after my brother and his family moved into their new home. The photographs we had seen didn't do the home and land justice. I've heard that a picture is worth a thousand words, but I was speechless.

My sister-in-law Julie is an amazing cook and baker. I'm not talking about someone who makes three or four recipes really well. I mean that Julie can whip up a restaurant quality meal on any given day. When she makes a big meal, she freezes some of it to provide for those times you fancy some home cooking, but don't have the energy to spend a lot of time in the kitchen.

My brother Will used his barbeque with pleasure. Julie and Chad's cooking styles blend well together.

We ate pitas stuffed with grilled turkey and fresh coleslaw on our first night there. Julie made a batch of pot stickers. Another night we had Swedish meatloaf. Will did up some pork chops on the grill.

For breakfast I craved a banana and nothing more. I usually slept late, so lunch wasn't an issue. I did eat a burger for a late lunch on the weekend we were in Napanee.

I didn't sleep as late as I sometimes do when I'm at home. Waking up to joyous kid noises is a fun way to ease into your day. Although once the children see your eyes are open, your sleep is done.

I slept on an aerobed in the family room near the toy area. I had a great sleep each night. I think that there have been some major improvements on the standard air mattress because I felt more comfortable than on my bed at home. Perhaps the mattress was the deluxe model.

*****

At Christmas time my mother would pick out age appropriate books for the little ones in our life. Now I get books for my nieces and nephews for no reason at all. I try to keep some on hand for surprise presents.

Zoe was my sidekick while we were in Napanee. She asked me to read a book to her on multiple occasions. She sees her parents reading and was curious as to how a person knows what is written on each page.

I was an adult before I read for pleasure. I read assigned books for school, but by the time my homework was done all I wanted to do was watch some mindless television.

One of my favourite activities to do is to sit around a fire pit and share stories. I was a fan of roasted marshmallows. I prefer mine to be a dark golden colour just before the fluff catches fire. Will toasts marshmallows to my specifications. He's the fire master at his house.

I got achy legs when I sit with my legs down for a long period of time. My legs were sore after riding in our minivan to Napanee with my feet down. A nice nap with the heating pad worked wonders.

Have you ever wondered if the weather gets chilly at night up north? Yes, the temperature gets colder than what I'm used to. Having the heating pad on my feet allowed me to fall into a deep sleep and stop moaning.

*****

Will and Julie had a small house warming party. We got to meet Nathaniel's parents and brother. Randy and Laurel Laughlin were so much like my folks. Nathaniel and Emily's youngest boy Sawyer was confused when his grandfather sat next to my Dad. Both men had gray hair and not much of it. They were wearing similar plaid shirts tucked into blue jeans.

Rumor has it that Laurel makes a great blue raspberry pie. I didn't know that blue raspberries were a real fruit. I thought that blue raspberries only existed in candies. Apparently the blue raspberries were in short supply that year, so there were only eight pies stored in the Laughlin's freezer.

Randy and Laurel brought date squares instead. They were yummy, but I was hoping to taste some real raspberry pie. Maybe next time. Until then, I'd munch on some blue raspberry skittles.

Inside Will and Julie's finished basement there was a wood stove for those cold winter nights, where all you did was curl up under a blanket. I look forward to cozying up to the fireplace.

*****

After Daphne and Jason had Cohen, they knew they had room in their hearts for more children. The two of them had a nice way of dealing with Cohen.

Daphne mentioned that they wanted more babies and a few months later she had a babe on board.

Little Chase was such a good little guy that Olivia and Eric considered adding another baby to their group. Eric and Liv were great with their little boy.

Liv and Eric didn't have to wait long for a passenger to climb aboard. They soon found out the little one was a boy.

Liv and Daphne didn't know one another, but they both were pregnant with baby number two at the same time.

Daphne and Jason had Briar Poppy in February of 2009. What a content babe they had. Briar was the audience for Cohen's one man show. He had a way about him that brought the house down night after night.

In August of 2009 Olivia and Eric had Maxwell Jacob Dickerson. Chase had a brand new person to read and share his toys with. For the first month or so Chase ignored baby Maxwell.

Everywhere I turned, infants and toddlers kept sprouting up. A few preschoolers thrown into the mix, to make life interesting.

*****

Food could wait. This was a day I'd recall forever. I broke free from my reverie to pay attention to what was happening around me at my university graduation.

Physiotherapy

Every student in the gymnasium has grown immensely since their freshman year. Some of us changed majors or decided on a different occupation.

*****

During September of 2008 I had begun intensive physiotherapy at a neurogym about ten minutes from our home. What the heck is a neurogym you might be asking? I had no clue until I got started. A neurogym is a physiotherapy clinic that is capable of dealing with patients who are having neurological issues. They have the equipment and specially trained staff.

I started to wake up to the smell of toast. My Mom had come in and tipped the blinds, allowing the sunlight to flood my bedroom.

Physiotherapy is something everyone anticipates they'll never make use of, but are glad it exists when they require some type of rehabilitation. I hadn't even had my first appointment.

I trusted Total Physiotherapy was as good as we'd heard they were. I was only asking them to do the impossible. If I ever hoped to walk again, I had to start somewhere. I didn't think walking was even on the table.

Francis Trolley would oversee my physiotherapy. He was an older man, in his early sixties, and spoke with a heavy Russian accent. He'd see me once a week for up to two hours. The therapists would push me to go further than I thought possible. Amelia Cortez, a kinesiologist in her mid-forties with long blonde hair in a ponytail, would also be on my team. The staff was committed to making a stronger version of me.

The initial assessment wasn't too bad, even though I was anxious. The people I'd be working with seemed nice. The mug sitting on the desk in the examining room scared me a bit. It read, "I don't like to repeat myself, so listen carefully".

I noticed that Francis was wearing dress socks and crocs. This was a fashion faux pas that I casually slipped into conversation when my Uncle Ted got a pair of the rubber clogs.

Francis knew his stuff, so how he dressed was irrelevant I suppose. Sometimes I surprise myself when I have a mature attitude about something. Besides, I have a pair of the rubber clogs for when we go in our pool area.

Don't get me wrong, I still see fashion mishaps now and then. I'm trying to lose the high school mentality, but that isn't as easy as you might think.

*****

Fall approached and the month changed to October. I was back at my physiotherapy gym for a workout. That day I'd be working with Ruby Valentia and Isaac Becker. Ruby was taking Frank's place from now on. She stood over five and a half feet tall; Isaac on the other hand was well over six feet.

I tried to wheel myself behind the curtained area, but when I got tired, Isaac pushed me. I started using the sit-to-stand equipment. I grabbed the handle bars, let my knees rest against the padding and slowly began to stand up. Isaac and Ruby were on either side of me and my wheelchair was behind me, so nothing was going to happen.

Isaac joked that they wouldn't let me fall more than once, which allowed my nerves to relax. I followed the instructions and stood up, my legs were shaking. Isaac beamed with pride, as a slight smile grew on my face. I did it. I was standing up... I had to sit down almost immediately, but for a brief moment I was upright. My parents noticed how tall I was when I stood up straight. Ruby wanted to have a look at my shoulder because Francis told her that it was achy from time to time.

Ruby wondered how I felt about needles. I wasn't a huge fan of the flu shot or blood work, but I still had needles without a problem. She was qualified to do acupuncture. The acupuncture needles are about 1/6th the size of the needle used to draw blood. Ruby thought that acupuncture, could improve the circulation in my legs and in turn make my feet warmer. Warm feet, a salty snack followed by a vanilla cupcake were key ingredients to a fun evening.

I craved poutine. We stepped outside onto the sidewalk where the smell of french fries wafted past our noses. I'd worked hard at physio, so I deserved a treat.

*****

I was ready for a workout. I was going to use the pulleys and small hand weights in addition to the sit-to-stand equipment. Ruby was prepared to try acupuncture on me, but only if I was sure I could handle it. Needles still made me nervous, but I was open to the idea.

Ruby began to clean between my toes. She used rubbing alcohol to sterilize the area, even though my feet were clean. Ruby began putting the miniscule needles in between each of my toes to increase my circulation. It sounded painful, but it wasn't as bad as I thought. She said that if at any time during the procedure I started to have funny or odd sensations, she would remove the needles. Sure enough, my toes began to warm once the needles were in place. Call it what you want, but my feet returned to a pink colour.

Winter was just around the corner. November began with the realization that I was about to get older. On Remembrance Day I turned twenty years old. My birthday wasn't an excuse to miss my physiotherapy time slot; exercising released endorphins.

Ruby was excited; she had me to use the pneumatic lift over top of the treadmill. They strapped me into a vest filled with compressed air which gave me the sense of being vertical. It was a fabulous way to create movement with my legs. Ruby had me do some lunges and marching.

Isaac put the treadmill on the slowest speed, but I couldn't keep up. Turning it on at any speed freaked me out a little. I'd seen those videos where somebody goes flying off the end of the treadmill. I laughed so hard I nearly peed. Isaac turned the treadmill off and I relaxed.

The vest reminded me of a jolly jumper that babies use. It's a more sophisticated design for adults, but a similar concept. I was all hooked in, not unlike a kid who was so bundled up in his or her snowsuit that he or she could barely move.

To keep my muscles loose, I did small exercises at home. I could see the benefits when I transferred from my wheelchair to the couch and vice versa. When I moved from my wheelchair to a seat in the minivan, I did more of the work myself.

The subsequent week, Ruby had a fresh idea for me to try. I'd be using the Nintendo Wii. Isaac set-up the gaming system, but I was confused as to how would I stand up. I used the pneumatic lift and the vest filled with compressed air to keep me in a standing position. I turned to face the television so that I could play balance games using the Wii Fit board.

Once I stood up, Isaac checked that all of the straps were securely done up. I used the treadmill hand grips to keep my balance while Isaac and Amelia attached the vest to the bar that was above me.

Amelia cheered me on as if I were an Olympian who'd just won a gold medal for Canada. I was thankful for her words of encouragement. Slalom skiing sounded like a fun activity. The object of the game was to shift my body weight from side to side to go through each set of flags. I had only seven misses on my first try, which was a great first run. Isaac hit the start button again and I flew out of the gates and down the hill. I had only four misses for my second attempt, which was a wonderful score.

I chose the river rafting in a bubble as my next game. This competition was similar to slalom with the side to side movements. I'd be travelling down a curvy river in a bubble. I had to watch out for the bees, they would burst my bubble with their stinger. A bumble bee came at me from nowhere and popped my bubble, so I had to race again. As it turns out, I was rather driven.

*****

On the ride home from my physio appointment, I got out my cell phone and began searching the internet to find out how much a Nintendo Wii gaming console cost. I found a Wii at Walmart and Costco. The system was over two hundred dollars and the balance board was another hundred dollars and that didn't include the sports resort game combo.

My parents agreed to buy the Wii and all of the games and accessories I would need. That would be a chunk out of my living money, so I was grateful. I'd talk to Isaac and Ruby next week and see if they thought a Wii would be beneficial for me to use at home.

*****

The New Year got here in a hurry. January was cold and wet, not exactly inspiring weather. I teased my parents as we crossed the parking lot toward the mall entrance, "Maybe exercising isn't so bad. After all, it gives me energy to go to more stores in the mall."

My Mom and I left my Dad at the news stand and headed down the mall to do our shopping.

Some cute workout attire was a must, so I didn't continually look like a slob at physio. I had to look presentable even when I was all sweaty. It didn't matter whether I desired to appear my best for Mateo Landry, a physiotherapist who worked with me from time to time.

As it turned out, I could do a lot of the balance games from my chair. It's a neat way to engage in exercise.

*****

Since Ruby was backed up with other patients, Mateo was dealing with me. My new yoga pants paid off. I got to work with Mateo. I'm pretty sure he had a girlfriend, but I could appreciate him from the sidelines.

The physiotherapists had me stand on a vibration plate. As I held the grab bars, the vibration stimulated my leg muscles. My physio routine was never dull.

My Mother flipped the calendar over to February of 2003. What a grey month. There was always a possibility of snow.

Ruby thought she should have a look at my shoulder in her exam room. She wheeled me in and I transferred to the massage table with the aid of her arms.

As Ruby manipulated my shoulder she informed me that she had another job. She couldn't tell me where it was because she didn't believe taking patients with her to her new clinic was right.

Ruby would be there for my next session, but after that Francis would step back in and be my head physiotherapist.

I kind of figured she'd be moving on soon. She took her physiotherapist training with Isla Layton, who used to live on my crescent. I heard that Isla got a promotion and a raise in pay, so I figured Ruby would be looking for a job with the possibility for advancement.

*****

I liked Francis alright, but I hoped he didn't take away my Wii time.

Time moved forward into March. The possibility of spring was on my doorstep.

My shoulder has been a bit crunchy, but not too much different than usual. Francis worked on my back and shoulder while I lay face down on the massage table.

Francis was closing a location on the mountain in two weeks. They were going down to two physiotherapy outlets. I'd continue to go to the Stoney Creek gym. It was great for me, because I lived about ten minutes from the new place. All of the neurogym equipment was moving too.

I was ready for some Wii action. Mateo pushed me toward the gym area. Since the clinic was moving and the harness and the pneumatic lift had been moved to another location temporarily, Mateo suggested using the parallel bars with the balance board between the bars.

I wasn't sure about my balance, but I gave it a chance. Mateo calmed my fears before I started. He said I wouldn't fall, he was right beside me and Isaac was on the other side. If I didn't see the benefits, I never had to do it again.

I took two steps forward and stepped on the balance board. Oh no. It was a lot harder to play sports on the Wii without the harness on. I didn't have a lot of balance to keep my body upright. I could always sit down because my wheelchair was behind me. I had only nine misses, which wasn't too bad for my first time without the vest on. I was bad on the Wii, but not as horrible as I had thought I'd be.

*****

The move in April went off without incident. All of my physiotherapy team worked at the Stoney Creek location. Amelia greeted my parents and me as we entered the new clinic location.

Mateo set me up on the vibration plate first. Amelia was on one side and he was positioned on the other side of me. Now that I was somewhat comfortable standing on the vibration plate, Amelia requested that I let one hand off of the grab bar. Mateo proposed that I release the other hand. They forced me to push beyond my limits.

I let go of both of the grab bars and it felt amazing. I was enjoying physio more than I thought I would. My Mom's eyes were misted with tears as we exited the clinic.

*****

I rolled in to the physio clinic and met Jude Coin. He was a physiotherapy student doing a placement at Total Physiotherapy. He'd be observing me during my session.

Mateo and Amelia thought I should learn to walk again, with assistance of course. I thought that they must have meant that I was going to move my feet while seated in my wheelchair. I was confused until I saw the masking tape line on the floor next to Mateo. I began to shake a little.

Mateo and Amelia supported my arms and I moved my feet along the line of tape. They had faith in me, but I wasn't sure that I believed in myself at this point.

I was panicking. I didn't have anywhere to go. If someone moved the wheelchair behind me as I walked, I would have been more confident. Mateo held my arm and Isaac stepped in to move the chair behind me as I walked.

Wow. Eight steps wasn't a lot, but it was for me. I couldn't believe I had walked.

My team of physiotherapists always had one more idea to try. We were never done.

Two more minutes on the vibration plate and my workout was done. Jude Coin was beside me, egging me on. I was getting tired, but the time wasn't over yet.

If Mateo were standing beside me, I'd be fine. Jude's dimples appeared upon his chubby cheeks. He had figured out that Mateo's attractiveness was a huge motivator. I knew he had a long term girlfriend, but I could still appreciate his beauty. Mateo had an outgoing personality.

I couldn't lie. Everybody had their own motivation.

Mateo was the perfect coach for me. He and Amelia worked well together, never letting me give up.

Each week the distance I walked grew by a few steps. Eventually I was able to walk without someone walking behind me with my wheelchair.

I was a rock star at my physiotherapy clinic. I'd likely never walk again without major assistance, but being upright felt fabulous.

One week my Dad made a video of me walking, so I could share my progress with close family and friends. I didn't care to have my videos ending up on YouTube or being shown over and over again.

My brothers and sisters-in-law were happy to see my progress. My brothers were excited that I was doing well. Will and Chad showed concern for my well-being without me feeling like they pitied me, because they didn't ever feel sorry for me.

I was proud of myself and all I had accomplished.

I continued walking with a physiotherapist on either side of me. Gradually the number of steps I took increased. Adding two or three steps each week didn't seem like much to me, but when I had a peek at one of the first videos my Dad had made tears filled my eyes at how far I had come.

*****

Weeks later I could do twenty-four steps in one direction and somehow manage to turn around and come back before collapsing in my wheelchair. Once I had rested for a bit, I stood-up and sat down about fifteen times. My work out sounds like it was designed by a person with obsessive compulsive disorder. But the repetitive actions were to build muscle memory.

With increased movement from me walking, I was experiencing a lot of pain in my lower back. My doctors increased my pain medication and had x-rays and scans done. The pain was likely from the end of the rods rubbing on bone. There was no guarantee that the pain wouldn't continue so they advised me to take a break and see how it went.

*****

I exuded so much effort to reach my goals. Now that I'm about to graduate from university I'll have to set out new objectives.

University Graduation

As the middle of May in 2010 grew closer, the due date for replying to graduation was itching closer. My dilemma was whether to go to my convocation or not. I wasn't sold on the idea of attending the ceremony because I used a wheelchair and I was nervous about being on stage.

If I chose not to go, then my family would support me. My Mom thought that I should explore my options before I decided what to do.

I wasn't sure what my options were. I was already stressed out about finishing my final university courses. My Dad suggested I email my advisor, Greta Kelley.

I hate when my parents make me choose without telling me what they think is the correct choice. I brought my arms to my lap.

I agreed to email Greta to discuss my situation. I wouldn't decide anything until I knew the facts. Does everything have to be a teachable moment?

Dear Greta,
I was wondering about graduation. Is it feasible for me to attend? I'm leaning toward not attending anyway, so if it isn't possible, that's alright.
If I do attend, is there a way for a family member to push me across the stage? I know that I couldn't wheel myself through the ceremony without assistance.
Thank you for all of your help.
Megan McIntyre

I sent Greta an email seconds ago. Why was I immediately expecting the doorbell sound that indicates that new email has arrived?

Hi Megan,
The last I heard, you were considering not going to your graduation. Have you decided yet?
I went to mine. It was long and hot, but in the end I'm glad I went. Graduation

is a rite of passage. Our speaker was a graduate who spoke about the book, "Oh the Places You'll Go" by Dr. Seuss. It was an interesting speech and not somebody droning on about meaningless crap.
I support your decision either way.
Olivia

Greta had a fulltime job before I wrote to her. I had to have a little patience.

Dear Megan,
Our graduation ceremonies are designed to be fully accessible and inclusive.
Don't for one minute think about not attending your own graduation. It is a big accomplishment and you deserve a moment in the spotlight. I will be attending your ceremony.
I've asked the graduation co-coordinator about you having a family member push you across the stage and he said that it'd be possible. If you send me the name of the person who will be wheeling you across the stage, I will fast track your paperwork and send you the pertinent information.
Take Care,
Greta Kelley

I asked my brothers and let them pick which one of them would push me. My mother's eyes became teary up at the thought of me attending graduation.

Daphne,
I'm going to attend university graduation! One of my brothers is going to wheel me across the stage.
My stomach is still full of jumping beans.
Megan

*****

Time passed until we reached October of 2010. My convocation date was fast approaching.

Megan,
I'm so proud of you.
You are amazing & we should celebrate that. How about we go to that dessert

place some Saturday?
Daphne

*****

I had better get a move on. October, 16th was my Graduation Day! My Mom flitted about, trying to get herself ready and keep everyone else on schedule. My Mom caught a glimpse of herself in the mirrored closet doors of our hall. She had forgotten to put earrings on.

My Mom put in my earrings that I was planning to wear. I thought I should wear the glittery white gold balls, but the backings were a real bastard to get on or off. I had trouble with earrings in general, so I never attempted to put on difficult studs.

I was totally ready. I finished spraying Lola perfume by Marc Jacobs, a graduation present from myself. To this day, if I smell that perfume, I think of my graduation ceremony. After all that rushing around we were all set to go early. That didn't happen often.

Was I ready to graduate? I was as ready as I'd ever be. That didn't mean I wasn't incredibly nervous. I hoped the ceremony would run smoothly. My parents told me that my feelings were normal. Will was going to be right by my side and he wouldn't let anybody bother me. Besides, everyone backstage was there to graduate.

Nobody would have thought twice if I'd packed my studies in early and didn't finish my degree. My Dad offered a hand to me and I held it. My family was super proud of me. I had to choose today of all days to wear mascara. I squeezed his hand.

I had to prove to myself that I could finish my degree despite my circumstances. I never felt pressure from anyone but myself to keep going. I have always been a stubborn person. I fight until I accomplish my goals.

We left before we had to so we would get to campus in time to drive around. The butterflies in my stomach were alive and well.

*****

My Dad paused in front of my residence building. My room looked occupied. Time had passed and yet the building exterior appeared as new as the day I moved in. The person in my room must have the desk under the window like I did, because I saw a Brock mug full of pens and highlighters.

The construction of the Life Sciences Building had started and completed in the time that I was taking online courses. Brock University was a growing campus that was constantly under construction.

The ceremony was in the modern glass fronted building. My Dad squinted into the sunlight as we walked toward the Walker Complex.

I sent Will a text telling him to meet us in the lobby of the new wing. I watched all of the guests and graduates flow through the main entrance.

My father gave Will a masculine hug. My sister-in-law Julie came with Will. Friends of my parents, Sadie Gregory and Logan Biker, were also waiting to take their seats in the audience.

Julie handed me a red rose, complete with baby's breath and a capsule of water to keep it fresh. How sweet was that?

Will was wearing La Coste cologne which smelled terrific! He looked fabulous in his navy suit. His tie was navy and red to match the school colours.

Will and I went to pick up my graduation gown. Julie stayed with our Mom and Dad. Will began to wheel me in the direction of the arrows on the wall.

Will was so proud of me. He even called me "baby". His eyes told me that tears of happiness nearly over flowed.

I managed to thank Will as I rapidly blinked back tears, hoping to avoid a mascara streak down my cheek. Will had many talents, but he wasn't a makeup artist.

I saw a sign as we entered the main foyer. I knew where to go now. We continued down a wide hall that had a gradual slope to the floor.

I gave my name to the ladies handing out the graduation gowns. I was told to ask for Robert Nighstrom when I arrived.

The lady said to find my place in line and she'd send Robert over to see me. The M section was in the far left corner of the gym.

Will tucked in the spare fabric so the excess material of my gown wouldn't catch in my wheels. I'd put on men's deodorant for the day. It tends to be stronger and on a special occasion the last thing I wanted was for my deodorant to fail.

Robert placed his arm on Will's shoulder. Introductions took place and then Robert began telling us how things were going to happen.

We'd come to the right man. Will tagged along with Robert so he could find out what route to take once we entered the ceremony area. Robert moved my guests up front so they could see the stage better.

As I took in my surroundings, the scent of a man wafted past my nose. Maybe I had a secret admirer who was afraid to approach me. Then again, it could have been my deodorant. What a letdown.

Greta was so glad I had decided to attend my graduation. She had pride in her eyes. Greta leaned over and hugged me just as Will returned. I introduced them to one another. I took a couple of deep breaths and tried to remain in a serene state. Greta had met the rest of my guests in the audience. She thought we had a beautiful family. Will thanked Greta for talking with Robert.

Greta said I was a special young woman. She took pleasure in creating a plan so I could reach my goals. She excused herself to take her seat in the gym. Greta slipped away, dabbing her eyes as she walked.

Will had a seat beside Julie and when it was time to move he'd come and get me. I thanked him for pushing me.

The ceremony was about to start. I was ready to roll! I gave Will two thumbs up and a big toothy grin. Robert had me to sit in the front row, so that I could see the events on stage. The bad news was that I had to at least appear to be paying attention because there was a photographer and videographer to my right.

The music started to play and the graduates began to file into the gym. "Pomp and Circumstance" was the tune. I hummed along.

The guy sitting next to me seemed so familiar. I wasn't meaning to sound like I was delivering a pick up line. I said he looked a lot like a Grant Charter. As it turned out, they were brothers. I was sitting beside Jeremy Charter.

Grant took dance lessons at the same studio as my best friend, Olivia Mason. I wouldn't be mentioning that Olivia referred to Graham as, Ginormous Grant. Some things are better left unspoken.

*****

The convocation speaker was Ingrid Flounder, a faculty member from the Child and Youth department, so I thought that she should be interesting.

The President of Brock University welcomed everyone to Fall Convocation 2010!

The only evidence that the ceremony space was a gymnasium was the basketball nets folded high in the rafters. I tried to take in all of the details that surrounded me.

*****

Ingrid Flounder took the microphone and placed her notes on the podium. She said when she was asked to be the convocation speaker; she was uncertain what to talk about.

When Ms. Flounder had been a student many years ago, she worked for a community organization that provided respite care to families of children with special needs. Ingrid indicated she learned a lot during those years and not just in her classes. The professor spoke clear and concise words.

Sometimes Ingrid would find the children she worked with in great moods and other times she'd walk in on a massive tantrum. Children, like life, could be unpredictable.

One day Ingrid arrived at a home and a little boy rolled a ball across the tile floor of the kitchen. She didn't realize until she got close to him that he played with a fecal ball.

I jumped back into the present and looked back at my family. Chad blinked his eyes to the sky. I had to look straight ahead on or I'd burst out laughing. We all had a sense of humour in my family and Chad uses his to get me laughing when I had to be serious.

Did she just say what I thought she said? I wondered if my graduation would be on YouTube.

I wanted my graduation to be memorable, but not because someone used the term fecal ball in the course of their speech. Did she think mentioning a fecal ball was appropriate for the occasion? Did she practice her talk with anyone? I doubted she'd rehearsed in front of family or colleagues because surely someone would have pointed her towards a more appealing topic.

Ingrid wished each graduate the best in all of their future endeavors. She hoped that as each student moved forward in life that we would always keep a piece of Brock University in our pocket. The audience clapped because she was finished speaking.

*****

The Master of Ceremonies pronounced my name into his microphone. With a smile plastered on my face, Will wheeled me across the stage. The Chancellor bent down to shake my hand and congratulated me. As I made my way across the stage I could hear the cheers from my family.

Chad noted the staff looked kindly at me. I was nervous to do the hand shake because my eye hand coordination wasn't one hundred percent.

*****

All of the late nights writing essays and studying faded into the background as my eyes flooded with tears of pure joy. A smile that simply wouldn't go away appeared when I received my degree.

Once we reached the hall my parents handed me a bouquet of flowers. I inhaled the heavenly smells of the red roses in my arms.

Sadie and Logan had to get my degree framed at the school store. There was a station with several rows of frames to choose from set up in the hallway.

I liked the cherry wood frame with the navy blue mat. I pointed to the frame and a staff member took my degree and frame to the back room to assemble it.

While Will and I waited for my degree to be framed my stomach gurgled in hunger. I hadn't eaten much before we left, so I was hungry for a solid dinner. Finally the line up at the framing station had died down.

*****

My parents met the rest of our party at a local restaurant for dinner and celebratory drinks. A steakhouse was a hit with our family and friends! I sniffed the smells of meat in the parking lot of a local dinner spot.

On our way into the restaurant, Chad and Nicole handed me a cookie bouquet. The cookies felt fresh. Yum! Chad knew how hard I worked for my degree. On top of the regular struggles that faced college and university students, I managed my time when I had online courses.

Before we ordered, Chad had us all laughing at the mention of a fecal ball. My convocation ceremony was a day we'd remember forever.

Everyone congratulated me! Someone made a toast saying, "Here's to a bright and beautiful future!" We clinked glasses and took a sip of our refreshments. I took a brief moment to admire my family. This day wasn't just about me. My family deserved some clapping!

*****

My former neighbour Addie found out that I hadn't seen the musical 'Wicked' and we planned a girl's night out with our mothers. The date that worked for all of us happened to be the Friday after my graduation ceremony.

We met for dinner before the musical. We arrived at our seats with only a moment to spare. Addie and Mia had seen the show several times before, but my mother and I hadn't been to a theatre performance in many years. The upbeat music impressed our ears. In fact, I bought the CD of the music and we listened to the songs on our way home.

*****

The following Saturday, my family and close friends were gathering in our condo social room to celebrate the hard work I had done in order to obtain my degree.

My brothers and their families assisted my parents in getting the party going. I didn't like that all eyes were on me. Eating cake when it wasn't a birthday or a wedding was an added treat. The food tasted particularly good at any McIntyre function. The fruit tray had watermelon and pineapple, both of which make my mouth water.

My best friend Olivia and her family came from Niagara. Olivia's husband Eric Dickerson came straight from his work as a stadium planner at a new sports complex in Hamilton. I was so touched that so many people came from other cities. Morgan came with her husband, Felix Westin.

The drop-in get together was a success. People came and had a glass of wine or punch and I visited with each guest. Each person was free to have a plate of sandwiches and dessert squares and stay awhile.

The afternoon went too fast for my liking. At times, I gazed at everyone in attendance and my eyes filled with tears. I now knew what it meant to be so happy you became weepy. As a small child I paused to wonder why an adult cried because their heart was exploding with joy.

*****

Dr. Sutton's words were stuck in my head. "Suck it up Sunshine!" I now understood what he meant. He didn't wish me to dwell on what I couldn't do. I had to figure out a way to do what was required to be done.

If I fell down, it was essential I find a way to pick myself up and continue on with life. Nobody promised life would be fair. With alterations my life would be what my dreams were made of. The cards you're dealt in the game of life didn't matter as much as how you played them.

I view the activities I couldn't do as a challenge. With a smile perfecting my face I'm ready to stare down whatever difficulties come my way.

I say to life, "CHALLENGE ACCEPTED"!

Epilogue

My parents named me Megan Heather McIntyre and my story didn't end because my book finished. My journey continued.

I checked an item off my bucket list. I wrote a book. It seemed impossible when I first started writing. A published author saw an untapped potential in me and gave me the necessary tools to write.

Some days I didn't write at all, while other days I wrote all afternoon. Every day had challenges and rewards; I just went with the flow. What did I do before I began writing a book?

Whether I wrote another book or not, I learned so much about myself. Through writing, all of my dreams were possible. I continued writing in some form or another. Whether I wrote a blog or online journal, I'd keep writing. I wouldn't trade the experience of writing my first book for the world.

Writing has assisted me in being a real adult. My friends have jobs or careers that kept them busy. Having a project with a goal brings a bit of normalcy to my life. Even though there wasn't a deadline or due date, I had the sense of being similar to every other thirty something.

I'd like Reese Witherspoon to play the adult version of me in the movie... Dream big. And the Oscar goes to...

Spending time with my nieces and nephew was one of my favourite activities to do. They bring a lot of fun with them wherever they go.

In the past I have said that children seemed to understand me better than some adults. While out to dinner with some extended family at a buffet restaurant, a friend's six year old daughter (who speaks another language and didn't understand much English) chose to sit beside me. We could only communicate through gestures and the odd word, yet we managed just fine.

Sabrina climbed up on my lap and played with my phone. She was comfortable enough to make herself at home with me. Children understand me, even without language skills.

Nature has a calming effect on me. You can talk if you wished, but scenery provides enough detail to keep my mind going for hours on end. I loved the beach. The idea of the ocean tides going out and coming in fascinated me. I see the waves as a metaphor for a fresh start.

Visiting my family in Napanee for the first time provided me with a great backdrop of inspiration. Even when I had a touch of pain in my legs, nature around me was enough to make me better.

Ten years ago I had no idea that I would be an author. I always thought I'd be working with little kids in some way. Circumstances meant my career ideas and plans had floated away. I adapted my future plans to fit my abilities. I didn't think of myself as different from other young adults. People adjust to roadblocks and move forward.

If I couldn't be a child life specialist, I was glad that Morgan could live out my dream. The children she works with were lucky to have such a mothering soul in their corner.

Morgan and I connected through residence, but have become forever friends. She changed my life for the better. We were neighbours first, but by the end of the year she was one of my best friends.

I learned to be flexible. Would I change my life if I could? Not a chance. Sure it would be nice to not have to worry about accessibility, but life was worth the challenges.

I met Daphne because of my disorder. I couldn't imagine my life without her. I didn't think we would have met if not for me having Friedreich's Ataxia. My disorder might be what brought us together, but it certainly wasn't the reason we remained friends.

I was comfortable with Daphne. She knows my medical history, so we don't have to talk about medical stuff I didn't want to. Daphne seemed to know when to avoid medical talk without me ever saying a word. She was a part of my family now and forever.

Olivia had been by my side through my ups and downs. I couldn't ask for a better friend. She never backed away from our friendship because I faced life in a wheelchair. I was grateful I had a best friend like Liv.

Norah had been my friends since I met her. Sometimes we go through periods of time where we didn't have much to say. When we did see one another conversation flowed. I had lots of cousins, but only one sister-cousin.

Some of my friend's children called me Auntie Megan. I'm honoured to fill that role. Regardless of what name they referred to me as, I would be there for them in any way I could.

I'd like a cure for Friedreich's Ataxia, so no one else had to endure the struggles that go along with the disorder. Life can throw me off balance, but it's my reaction to adversity that will decide whether I'm miserable or happy. I choose to look for positivity in the most unlikely places.

I could decide to be morose about my situation in general, but that doesn't allow for fun times to animate my days. Life isn't going to be rewarding if every time you hit a pot hole you crawl back into the dark and merely exist. My Dad's father gave him that piece of advice when he was on the cusp of adulthood. When I'm feeling down, I can pull out that memory file in my head. I never met my Grandpa McIntyre, so to be able to carry his advice in my pocket means a lot to me.

Honestly, I'd like to get married and have children. If a guy doesn't desire me as is, then I sure as shit won't let him in my life when I'm well. And I definitely won't be the mother of his children.

My name is Megan McIntyre, thank you for joining me on the ride that is my life. I learned to hold on tight because the road might get bumpy, but that adds to the experience.

About the Author

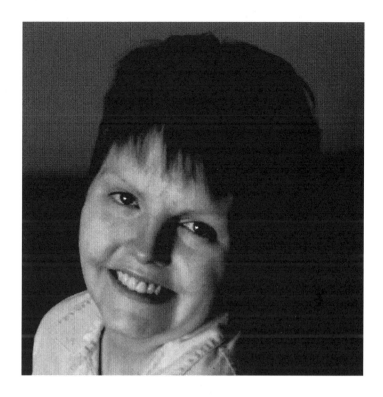

My name is Megan McIntyre and I am a thirty-four year old daughter, sister, granddaughter, niece, cousin, aunt, friend and now author. I was diagnosed with a neuromuscular disorder called Friedreich's Ataxia (F.A.) at age fourteen. F.A. is a part of me, but I won't let my illness define who I am.

I could have chosen to be blue after my diagnosis, but I prefer be optimistic whenever possible. My positive attributes highlight what I can do, as opposed to what I am not capable of doing. I refuse to be held back.

My degree in Psychology has facilitated a greater understanding of my emotional self. No two people are exactly alike and therefore each human approaches the world differently.

Because I fight for everything I do, I appreciate when a simple task goes well. I'm stubborn by nature, so giving up was never an option I considered.

Contact: meganmcintyreauthor@gmail.com